Latch Baby

Illustrated Guide to Breastfeeding Success

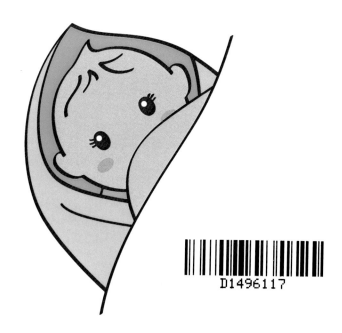

D1496117

Tracey Jedrzejek, MA, IBCLC
Illustrated by Bridget Halberstadt

Latch Baby
Illustrated Guide to Breastfeeding Success
Copyright © 2019 by Tracey Jedrzejek
Designed and Illustrated by Bridget Halberstadt
Edited by Audrey Kalman

Printed in the United States of America
First Printing, 2019
First Edition
ISBN-13-978-0-692-18695-4
Visit www.traceylactation.com

TABLE OF CONTENTS

INTRODUCTION

Breastfeeding is the normal and natural way to feed human babies. New moms who want and plan to breastfeed are often surprised to learn that the natural way to feed their babies doesn't always feel so natural. You may be reading this book as a pregnant mom, committed to giving breastfeeding a try, but feeling nervous and unsure about whether you will be successful. Or you may have given birth already and are seeking information because breastfeeding isn't going as smoothly as you had hoped. Perhaps a friend happily breastfed her baby till he was four years old, but another friend was in so much pain that she quit after the first week. Or maybe your sister wanted to breastfeed her baby but wasn't able to make enough milk. All of these are very legitimate concerns! Good for you for seeking out resources like this book to help support you right from the start.

For many women, being able to breastfeed is one of the most rewarding joys of their lives. Yet, for many new mothers, breastfeeding is challenging in the beginning as they-and their babies!-learn this new skill. The good news is that most women can successfully breastfeed, providing their babies with the nourishment and comfort they need to grow and develop. With some knowledge, support, and perseverance, you can develop an incredible bond with your baby while enjoying the ease of being able to offer her the best possible nourishment anytime and anywhere.

My first breastfeeding experience went smoothly despite a thirty-one-hour labor. My daughter latched right away and continued breastfeeding for almost a year. Although I had some initial soreness, it didn't last long as my daughter and I learned together. My son was also a good breastfeeder but the nipple soreness continued throughout the first month. I called my pediatrician and she put me in touch with a lactation consultant who came to my home. She helped me adjust the latch, the soreness decreased, and we were able to enjoy breastfeeding for more than a year. I am so grateful that I needed a lactation consultant, despite not knowing what one was, as my experience with her encouraged me to become a lactation consultant myself!

As a lactation consultant in private practice in Silicon Valley, I have helped hundreds of moms and babies breastfeed successfully. I wanted to create a book full of practical advice and beautifully clear illustrations to share my knowledge with you in a simple and non-judgmental way. My hope is that this book will help you feel supported and empowered throughout your breastfeeding journey. You can do this!

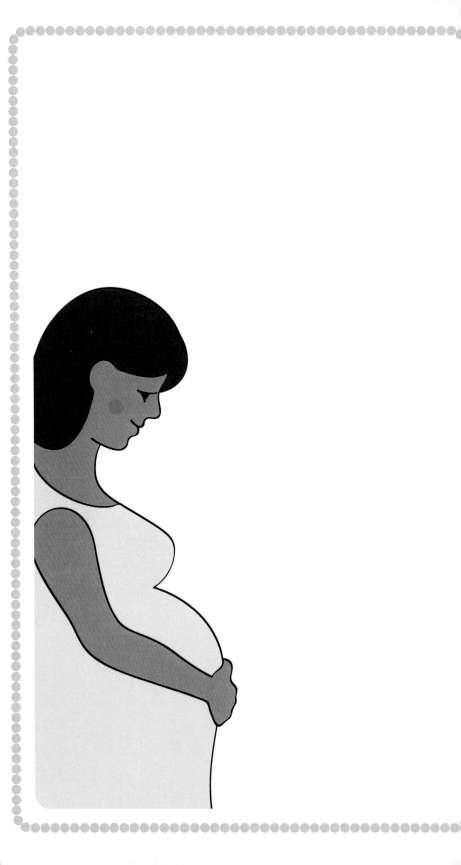

CHAPTER 1
BEFORE BABY ARRIVES

Congratulations on your pregnancy! If you are reading this book, you have taken the first step toward providing your baby with the most natural, complete, and superior source of nutrition. Educating yourself and your partner about breastfeeding during your pregnancy can help you to feel prepared and comfortable right from the start.

BENEFITS OF BREASTFEEDING

You may have already heard about the numerous benefits of breastfeeding. Here are just a few:

Benefits for Baby

- Easily digested, designed specifically for your baby at each age/stage
- Promotes secure bonding with mom and soothing comfort for baby
- Contains hormones and growth factors essential for growth
- Supports oral and motor development
- Aids in ensuring a strong immune system
- Lowers the risk of obesity
- May reduce the risk of developing diabetes and allergies
- May reduce the number of upper respiratory infections

Benefits for Mom

- Easy preparation (always warm and available)
- Quality time to bond with baby
- Lowers risk of developing certain health conditions (postpartum depression, breast and ovarian cancer, Type 2 diabetes)
- Reduces amount of postpartum bleeding
- May contribute to faster postpartum weight loss

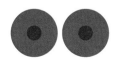

Benefits for Family/Community

- Zero financial cost
- Lower healthcare costs due to less illness
- Fewer days lost from work to care for sick baby
- No environmental consequences (nothing manufactured and no waste)

BREAST ANATOMY

Breasts come in many different sizes and shapes. Some are extremely large and some quite small, some are round and some are more pointy. Some women even have a right breast that looks completely different from their left! Regardless of their breast size and shape, most women are able to successfully breastfeed.

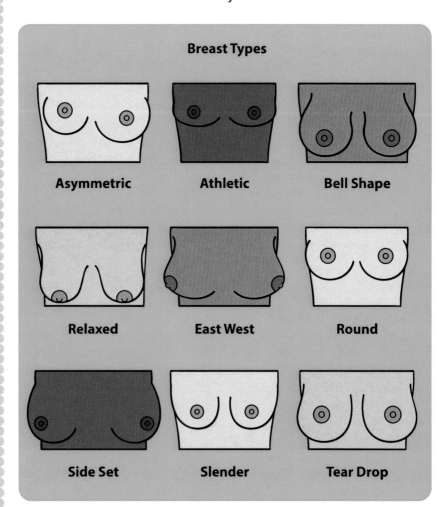

Breast Types

Asymmetric | Athletic | Bell Shape

Relaxed | East West | Round

Side Set | Slender | Tear Drop

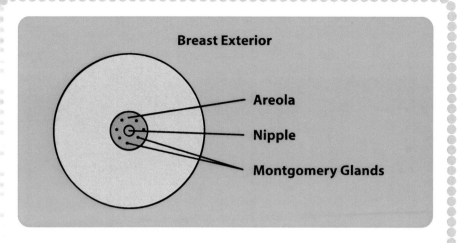

Breast Exterior

Breast Exterior

The outside of mom's breast consists of the areola and the nipple.

Areola

The areola is the darker, circular area surrounding the nipple. It contains small bumps called Montgomery glands that secrete an antibacterial oil that helps soothe the areola and nipple. Some believe this oil contains a scent that helps baby find the breast. These glands may not appear during pregnancy but typically become more prominent once baby is born.

Nipple

Each nipple contains approximately 9 to 15 pores for milk to flow through. Just like breasts, nipples come in all shapes and sizes. Some nipples are flat and some are protruding. Some are large and some small. Most moms can breastfeed regardless of the size or shape of their nipples. However, if you have inverted, flat, or very large nipples, it's best to work with a lactation consultant right from the start to ensure optimal latching and milk transfer.

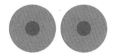

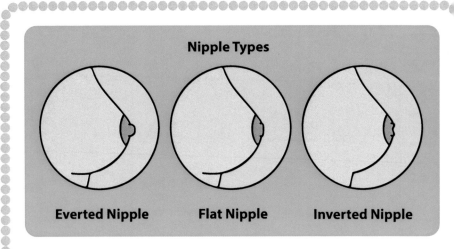

Nipple Types

Everted Nipple   Flat Nipple   Inverted Nipple

Nipple Types

Everted: nipple extends outward from the areola
Flat: nipple does not extend outward from the areola
Inverted: nipple extends inward, but can usually be pulled out
with suction

Breast Interior

The interior breast tissue contains glands that make breastmilk and
ducts that transfer milk to the nipple. Surprisingly, breast size has little
to no influence on mom's milk supply. Instead, it is the amount of
interior mammary glands/tissue that determines mom's milk
production and storage capacity. Therefore, having large breasts does
not necessarily mean you will have a copious milk supply. The amount
of milk produced varies among women and even per breast.
Interestingly, many moms produce more milk in the right breast than
the left.

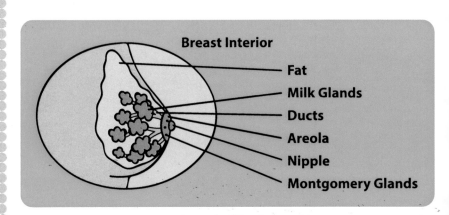

Breast Interior

Fat
Milk Glands
Ducts
Areola
Nipple
Montgomery Glands

Breast Changes During Pregnancy

Many women experience breast changes during pregnancy as their bodies prepare for baby's arrival. One of the most common changes is nipple sensitivity during the early weeks of pregnancy as your milk-making cells begin to grow. In fact, for many women, this is one of the earliest signs of pregnancy. During pregnancy, most women's bra band size increases as their ribs expand to help carry the weight of the baby, and most women's breasts grow bigger by about one cup size. Veins on the breasts may become more visible due to the increased blood flow during pregnancy. Your areola may become darker and the Montgomery glands on your areola may become more pronounced. Your breasts typically will double in size during the first few weeks after birth but eventually will return to their pre-pregnancy size. Toward the end of pregnancy, your breasts may leak a little of the first milk, called colostrum.

My boobs are leaking something orange!

I will never forget the text I got from a mom during her eighth month of pregnancy. It read: "Help! My breasts are leaking something orange!" I assured her that she was simply leaking colostrum, baby's first milk, which appears yellow or orange in color. It is perfectly normal to have some leakage of colostrum toward the end of your pregnancy. But don't worry if you don't see it-it's still there, ready to feed your baby when she's born!

PREPARATION FOR BABY'S ARRIVAL

There is absolutely nothing you *need* to do to prepare for breastfeeding before your baby is born. However, here are some things you might want to take care of before your baby arrives.

Inform your obstetrician or midwife of your plans to breastfeed.

This will help to ensure minimal separation from your baby after the birth. If you've had previous breast surgery of any type (implants, reduction, biopsy), let your obstetrician or midwife know and contact a lactation consultant before baby arrives. That way you will have your support team in place to address any supply issues right from the start. For more information regarding breastfeeding after breast surgery, visit BFAR (www.bfar.org).

Find a pediatrician who is supportive of and knowledgeable about breastfeeding.

This will help to ensure you get the support you and your baby need throughout your breastfeeding journey.

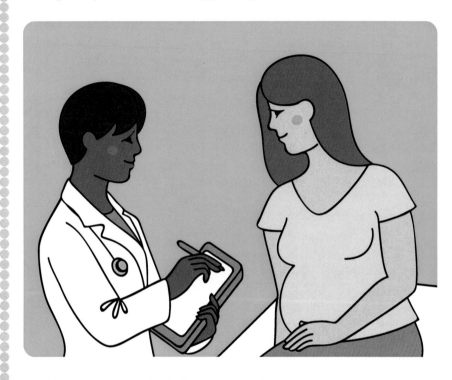

Decide where you will deliver your baby.

Most moms deliver in a hospital, but you also have the option of delivering your baby at a birthing center or at home. This is a personal decision for you and your partner to make together. If you are planning to deliver your baby in a hospital, look for one with the designation of Baby-Friendly (www.babyfriendlyusa.org). The designation of Baby-Friendly is given by the World Health Organization and UNICEF to hospitals that are committed to providing the highest standard of infant care while encouraging the mother/baby bond. If your local hospital is not designated as Baby-Friendly, ask about their policy on rooming in and on skin-to-skin contact directly after birth. Also find out about their in-hospital lactation support and what breastfeeding support they offer once you head home with your baby. Many hospitals provide weekly breastfeeding support groups that you can attend with your baby.

Check with your insurance company regarding lactation visits and pump purchases.

Most insurance companies cover lactation support and pump rentals or purchases, but it's a good idea to call your insurance company ahead of time and ask about your particular plan's coverage. If you are required to see a lactation consultant who is within your insurance company's network of providers, ask whom you can see in your area. If the insurance company cannot provide the name of an in-network local lactation consultant, ask if you can see the lactation consultant of your choice at 100% coverage. Some insurance companies will provide you with a breast pump free of charge. Ask about the different pump options so you can research them ahead of time. If you are returning to work, ideally you will want a double electric breast pump.

Do some research on local lactation consultants.

The most knowledgeable and experienced lactation consultants have earned the degree of IBCLC (International Board Certified Lactation Consultant), and these initials should appear after their names. These professionals have completed many clinical and classroom hours and have passed a medical board exam. When contacting an IBCLC, ask if she comes to the hospital or your home, how much she will charge, and whether she accepts insurance. Find out how much time she allows per visit (most provide one to two hours) and ask if the visit

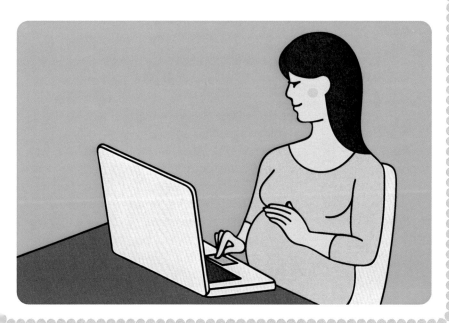

includes ongoing email and/or text follow-up support. You can find referrals to local lactation consultants through your hospital or birthing center, your obstetrician, your pediatrician, and online at ILCA (www.ilca.org).

Attend a prenatal breastfeeding class with your partner or a support person.

These classes are offered through local hospitals or childbirth education centers. The information you learn will be helpful once baby arrives. If possible, attend a breastfeeding support group meeting, such as those offered by La Leche League (www.llli.org), while pregnant. There, you can witness other moms breastfeeding and listen to their experiences. Also, those moms will be there to support you once your baby arrives.

Join a local mothers'/parents' club.

Search for clubs in your area and check out their websites ahead of time. You can often join a playgroup through the club for babies born around the same time as yours. Most playgroups have an online chat forum and weekly playdates at a member's house or at a park. These clubs are a great way to meet new parents and bounce ideas off each other as you navigate through the new world of parenting. Plus, your baby will get lots of social interaction as she grows and develops new friendships.

Think ahead about visitors.

Give some thought ahead of time about when you will accept visitors once baby has arrived. Ideally, your loved ones will wait for an invitation to come meet the baby, but some might arrive without being invited. This can be disruptive to your new routine with the baby and can interfere with you getting enough rest. If you are delivering in a hospital, you may not want visitors to come into the room until you have had a few hours alone with your new baby and your spouse/partner. If you desire this private time, tell your loved ones ahead of time that you will let them know when you are ready for visitors. You will never get this precious time alone with your newborn again, so don't feel shy about setting firm boundaries. You also may want to inform the nursing staff in the hospital of your wishes so they can help you advocate for the privacy you desire.

Privacy, please!

I remember visiting a mom in the hospital the day after her baby's birth. She had a room full of visitors, including her dad, and she didn't have the heart to ask her family to leave the room while we worked together on breastfeeding. It would have been nice for us to have some privacy during the consultation so she could relax and focus on learning to feed her baby. After the session, she shared with me that she wished she had been more assertive about asking for privacy.

BREASTFEEDING ITEMS FOR YOUR HOSPITAL BAG

These are a few things you might consider bringing to the hospital to ease your breastfeeding experience, though none of these is mandatory for initial breastfeeding success.

Breastfeeding Pillow

Pillows help to ensure correct positioning and latch while supporting you and your baby during the early weeks of breastfeeding. You can bring your own breastfeeding pillow to the hospital or use the hospital bed pillows during your stay. There are many different brands of breastfeeding pillows. The best ones are firm enough to support the weight of your baby in the correct position and provide back support for you while breastfeeding. My favorite breastfeeding pillow is called My Brest Friend (www.mybrestfriend.com).

Nursing Bras

Many moms want the support of a nursing bra 24 hours a day in the early weeks of breastfeeding. You will want to buy a few bras that are supportive yet soft and stretchy, allowing for breast size changes and frequent feedings in the first two weeks postpartum. Make sure that the bra is not too tight or binding (sports bra) or too rigid (underwire), which can restrict milk flow and cause plugged milk ducts. There is no need to purchase a fitted nursing bra until your milk supply regulates a bit, around 2-1/2 weeks postpartum. At this time, you may also want to purchase some nursing tank tops you can wear in place of a nursing bra. These tanks are comfortable and cover your abdomen while you're breastfeeding. One company that makes terrific nursing bras is called Kindred Bravely (www.kindredbravely.com).

Nipple Creams

There are many brands of nipple creams on the market that you can apply to your nipples after feedings. These can be very soothing during the early days of breastfeeding. My favorite product for soothing nipples is coconut oil. It is natural, has healing properties, and you can purchase it at your local grocery store. Breastmilk itself has antibacterial and antimicrobial properties, and some moms like to manually express a small amount of breastmilk and rub it into their nipples after breastfeeding, instead of using creams or oils.

Breast Pads

Some moms find it helpful to have a barrier between their bra and nipples during the initial weeks of breastfeeding. Breast pads work to collect any leaking milk, help prevent staining of your bra from nipple creams, and help to hold breasts in place to avoid chafing of your nipples. You can purchase either washable/reusable or disposable pads. If you use washable pads, 100% cotton with no plastic lining are best, to improve breathability. Change breast pads frequently and anytime they feel moist to prevent an overgrowth of yeast or bacteria.

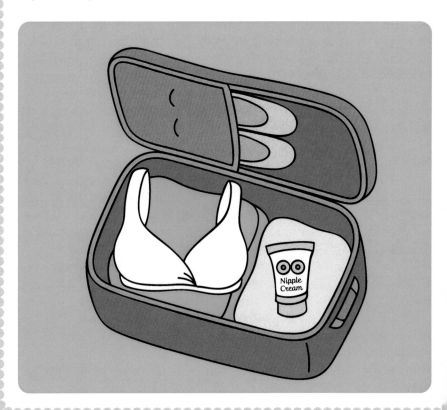

CHAPTER 2
BREASTFEEDING AFTER BABY ARRIVES

Congratulations! Your baby has arrived. Now that you have given birth, it's time to focus on your next main responsibility . . . breastfeeding!

Skin to Skin

Directly after birth, your baby should be placed on your bare chest. She will feel comforted by your exclusive scent, your familiar voice, and your heartbeat, just as she was for the previous nine months. Holding her skin to skin will help regulate her body temperature and her heart rate. There is no rush to weigh and bathe your newborn; you can request that the hospital staff delay routine procedures for an hour or two. This initial bonding time is so important for both of you. Partners can also do skin to skin with baby.

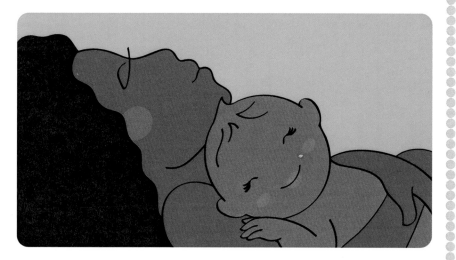

Can I please hold my baby?

I remember thinking it was strange that directly after the birth of my daughter, she was across the room, lying alone in a warming bed, when she could have been staying warm in my arms, being comforted by me. I wish I could go back in time and insist that she stay with me directly after the birth.

First Latch

If possible, breastfeeding should be initiated within the first hour after birth, when babies are often awake and alert. Amazingly, if held skin to skin right after birth, many babies use their natural instincts to find the breast and latch on by themselves within the first hour. Other babies need a little help from mom and the postpartum support team. If your baby does not seem ready to latch, hold her close, skin to skin, and gently try again after some time has passed. Look for signs of readiness, such as turning her head toward your chest or opening her mouth. It's never a good idea to force a baby to latch on to the breast.

Rooming In

Ideally, mom and baby should remain in the same room during the postpartum period to encourage a strong breastfeeding relationship. This way, mom can respond quickly to baby's hunger cues, encouraging a healthy milk supply and a strong mom-baby bond. If you need to be separated after the birth for medical or other reasons, try to spend as much time with your baby as possible. If your baby is in the hospital nursery, ask the nurse to call you for feedings when your baby wakes up and at least every three hours around the clock.

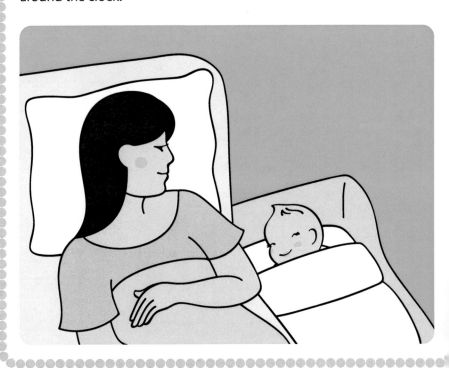

Hospital Support

If you deliver your baby at a hospital, a nurse will be assigned to you who can help with postpartum care, baby care, and breastfeeding. Keep in mind that the amount of breastfeeding education nurses receive varies and can be limited. Although they have every intention of supporting you, they may not have the knowledge and experience of a lactation consultant. A common complaint from postpartum moms is that everyone at the hospital told them something different when it came to breastfeeding. I encourage moms to ask to see a lactation consultant as soon as possible. She can teach you tips and tricks based on her experience and continued training as you and your baby learn to breastfeed.

Frequent Feedings

It is important to feed your baby on demand during these first few weeks, which means feeding her anytime she is awake and wants to suck. You'll want to make sure she is breastfeeding at least every three hours, measured from the start of one feeding till the start of the next feeding, around the clock. This translates to 8 to12 times or more in a 24-hour period. Many babies cluster feed, which means they feed at intervals much closer than every three hours before taking longer breaks. You may feel like all you are doing is breastfeeding! Just remember that these frequent feedings will help to ensure that your baby gets the nutrients and calories she needs while bringing in a healthy milk supply. The time your newborn spends breastfeeding can vary from 5 to 30 minutes at each breast in the beginning, so be sure to watch your baby and not the clock. A tip for rousing a baby who is sleepy at the breast is to undress her, leaving the diaper on. Ensuring that baby is not overly warm can help keep her awake and being skin to skin with you will regulate her temperature. You can also lay her flat on a blanket, which wakes most newborns if they are not swaddled. Look for large jaw movements and a continuous sucking pattern versus a slower and more irregular pattern that signifies comfort sucking. It is perfectly fine to allow your baby to comfort suck, even after she has transferred enough milk. When baby begins to suck less consistently, you can squeeze your breast to see if she will eat more. If she continues comfort sucking for a few more minutes, falls asleep, or comes off the breast on her own, you can assume she is done on that side. Try burping her for a few minutes before offering the second side. During these early weeks, try to feed your baby on both breasts at each feeding session to stimulate your milk supply. Also, it's important to alternate which breast you start feedings on.

Milk Supply and Hormones

Many moms wonder if they have any milk for their baby in the first few days. Actually, your body has been making milk since the second trimester of your pregnancy! The hormones prolactin and oxytocin work together to make milk. The delivery of the placenta triggers the release of prolactin, which tells your body to increase your milk supply. Oxytocin is responsible for releasing the milk when a baby sucks at the breast, a process called letdown. As your baby demands milk often, your breasts will continue to make milk and increase your supply. Although you probably won't feel any breast fullness for the first few days if it's your first baby, your milk supply should significantly increase in volume (sometimes referred to as "milk coming in") by day four. It may take a day or two longer after a cesarean birth, and often takes a shorter amount of time if this is not your first breastfed baby.

I don't have any milk!

I'll never forget what happened in the hospital shortly after the birth of my daughter. I squeezed my breast, expecting milk to come out, and when that didn't happen, I yelled to my husband, "Go get the nurse and tell her that I don't have any milk!" The nurse came in and quickly assured me that I indeed had milk but that because the milk volume is so low in the beginning, milk would not come shooting out of my breast from one little squeeze. Phew!

Colostrum

The first milk that your baby will drink is called colostrum. Colostrum contains powerful antibodies that protect baby's immature immune system, lining her tummy to seal and protect it against any foreign bacteria. It is high in protein and low in sugar and fat. Colostrum is thicker than mature milk and lower in volume to help baby learn to suck, swallow, and breathe while

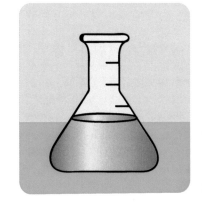

breastfeeding. It is also a natural laxative that helps baby to poop. Many people refer to colostrum as "liquid gold" because it is so high in nutrients. The yellowish/orange color (hence "gold") is caused by the presence of beta-carotene, which is known to be a powerful immune system protector.

High Suck Need

Although babies do not typically feel hunger in the first few days of life, they will act like they want to eat often because they are born with a high suck need. This high suck need helps to stimulate mom's milk supply after birth. Regular breast stimulation of at least every three hours around the clock helps to increase mom's milk supply to meet baby's needs. Another reason babies are born with a high suck need is to stimulate their tummies to eliminate the first poop, called meconium. Meconium is sticky, tarry, and black, and is the product of baby ingesting mom's amniotic fluid in the womb.

Trouble Latching

Sometimes babies struggle to latch during their first few days of life for a variety of reasons. The problem might be something minor such as poor positioning or something more challenging like an anatomical issue. As a new mom, your main focus when nurturing your baby will be to feed her. If your baby isn't latching, you might feel discouraged or even rejected. These feelings are normal, but do not despair! Remember, this is a learned skill, and most babies will latch eventually. Seek the help of a lactation consultant or your nurse/midwife as soon as you can to help your baby to latch. If your baby is not latching regularly (about every three hours), it will be extremely important for you to feed her using an alternative feeding method. In addition, you will need to protect your milk supply with breast stimulation until your baby is ready to do this on her own. Continue lots of skin-to-skin contact, which will encourage your baby's natural instinct to breastfeed and will help stimulate your hormones to continue making milk.

Manual Expression of Colostrum

If your baby is not latching regularly after birth, you can provide nourishment for her by using your hands to remove colostrum. Try to do this once every hour until your baby is latching frequently.

To manually express colostrum from your breasts:

- Place your thumb and index finger in a C shape about a half inch away from your nipple on either side.
- Press in toward your chest wall.
- Compress your areola by squeezing your thumb and finger toward each other.
- Let go of the compression and repeat continuously for about five minutes per breast. You may need to experiment to find the right spots to compress.
- Express colostrum into a spoon or small container.
- Feed colostrum to your baby using a spoon, syringe, or small cup.
- Repeat this process as often as possible until your baby is ready to latch regularly.

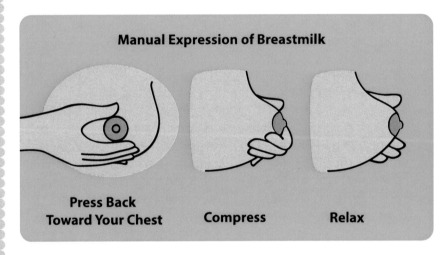

Manual Expression of Breastmilk

Press Back Toward Your Chest   **Compress**   **Relax**

Pain with Breastfeeding

Breastfeeding is not supposed to hurt if your baby is latching on correctly. However, learning to breastfeed takes time and practice. It can be challenging to get your newborn to open her tiny mouth wide enough to get a deep latch in the early days. Even if your baby latches correctly, you may experience some initial soreness from the sheer number of hours per day that your newborn will be sucking on your breasts. Therefore, it does take some getting used to. If you are experiencing a lot of pain that is not getting better, reach out to a lactation consultant for help as soon as possible. If continuing to breastfeed is too painful, you will need to extract milk using a double electric breast pump to protect your milk supply.

Pumping to Protect Your Supply

If the latch is too painful or your baby isn't latching regularly, you will need to pump both breasts often to protect your milk supply. Use a hospital-grade pump versus a personal pump during these early weeks. If you gave birth in a hospital, the nurse or lactation consultant can provide you with a hospital-grade breast pump for use during your stay. You can then rent one to take home with you, either from the hospital or a local breastfeeding center. The general protocol is to pump both breasts at the same time every three hours for fifteen minutes. You can feed any pumped milk to your baby with a spoon, cup, or syringe. Check with your pediatrician or lactation consultant about appropriate amounts of milk to give to your baby.

Low Milk Volume

Remember that the amount of milk you pump will be low during these early days. This is not an accurate indication of how much milk you actually have. Your body does not release milk for a breast pump as easily as it does for your baby. Even if you are not getting any milk initially, make sure you continue pumping every three hours for the full fifteen minutes. The breast stimulation alone will tell your body that it should continue making milk. Feed any milk collected to your baby using a spoon, syringe, or small cup. It is best not to introduce a bottle at this point until breastfeeding is well established, usually at about four weeks. Continue regular skin-to-skin contact with your baby in addition to pumping.

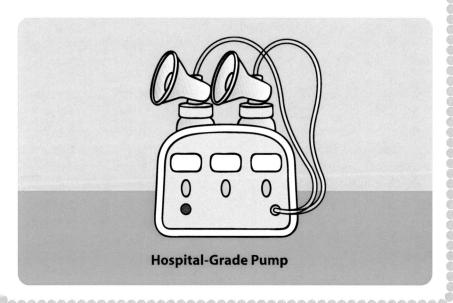

Hospital-Grade Pump

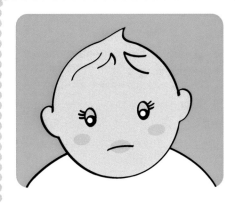

Jaundice

Frequent feedings help to prevent jaundice, a common condition in newborn babies that can appear within the first few days of life. Jaundice is caused by a build-up of bilirubin (red blood cells) that is not being excreted through baby's stool fast enough.

Sucking stimulates your baby to poop, which is why frequent feedings are encouraged in the first few days of life. Baby's skin and the whites of her eyes may appear yellowish when baby is jaundiced. Jaundice typically peaks on the fifth day of your baby's life and usually resolves on its own through frequent feedings. As the jaundice decreases, the yellowish color will gradually fade from your baby's feet, moving up to her face before completely resolving.

Pumping in the First Month

There is no reason to begin pumping during the first four weeks after birth unless your baby is not latching or you are giving a supplement (formula or donor milk) in addition to or in place of breastfeeding. Each time your baby removes milk from your breasts, your body gets programmed to continue making that amount of milk for your baby. If you regularly pump after feedings in the first few weeks, your body may think you have twins and will make more milk than your baby needs. This can cause tummy upset for your baby and may cause a breast infection. Therefore, it's best to continue breastfeeding on demand and let your baby program your body on her own.

Pacifiers

Pacifier use within the first four weeks after birth is not recommended for breastfed babies as it can interfere with breastfeeding. Although newborns have a high suck need, ideally, when they want to suck, they should be sucking on mom's breast, stimulating her growing milk supply. When baby sucks on a pacifier, she builds muscles that encourage a shallow latch when at mom's breast. A shallow latch can be extremely painful for mom and can decrease mom's milk supply. It's best to wait about four weeks or until breastfeeding is established before introducing a pacifier.

Pacifier Refusal

My first child absolutely loved her pacifier and used it for two years. Once breastfeeding was established, it became a comforting tool for her when she was going to sleep or when she was upset. I introduced a pacifier to my second child once breastfeeding was established, assuming he would love it too. After trying numerous different pacifiers, he never took to one. It's true what they say: every baby is different.

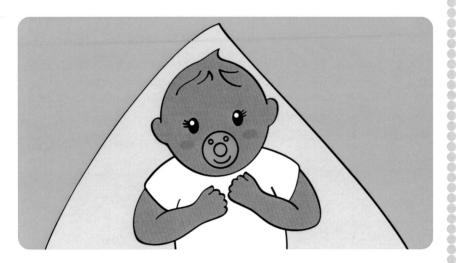

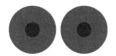

CHAPTER 3
POSITIONING AND LATCH

Obtaining a good latch is one of the most important things you can do to prevent sore nipples and ensure that your baby gets enough milk. However, it isn't always easy in the first few days and weeks. You and your baby will learn together, but seek help sooner rather than later if you're having trouble getting your baby to latch or are experiencing pain while feeding.

Breastfeeding Station

During the early weeks, it's a good idea to establish a place in your home where you will typically breastfeed, so you have all of your supplies handy. As you become more comfortable with breastfeeding, you will find yourself feeding your baby in any room of the house and while you are out and about, with or without supplies.

Recommended supplies for your breastfeeding station:

- Water for mom
- Snacks for mom
- Breastfeeding pillow
- Extra pillows
- Burp cloths
- Nipple cream/oil
- Smartphone, tablet, or notebook

Breastfeeding Logs or Apps

At your first few pediatrician appointments, the doctor will likely ask you about the number of feedings and diaper changes per day. You can log this in a notebook, though many parents enjoy tracking this data using a smartphone or tablet app. These apps track the number of feedings, which side mom fed on and when, the number of pees and poops, and the color of the baby's poop at diaper changes. This information will be important to know in the first few weeks to remind you which breast you last fed on and to ensure that breastfeeding is going well. After the first

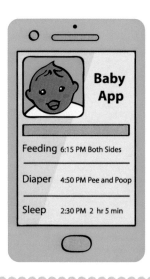

Baby App

Feeding 6:15 PM Both Sides

Diaper 4:50 PM Pee and Poop

Sleep 2:30 PM 2 hr 5 min

few weeks, you won't need to track this information if your baby is eating frequently, peeing and pooping regularly, and gaining an appropriate amount of weight. Some of the most popular baby care apps are Baby Connect and Baby Tracker.

Pillows

Before settling down to start a feeding, you'll want to set up your pillow or pillows to help support you and your baby. Any pillow can work, but the pillows that are made specifically for breastfeeding do an effective job of positioning your baby at breast height while also supporting you and your baby's body. Use as many pillows as you need to support your baby at breast height so you don't have to hunch over. Some moms appreciate having a pillow behind their back for support, especially if sitting in a deep chair or couch. Make sure there are no gaps between the pillow and your body. Whatever setup you use, the goal is to make sure you can completely relax once the baby latches. My favorite breastfeeding pillow is called My Brest Friend (www.mybrestfriend.com).

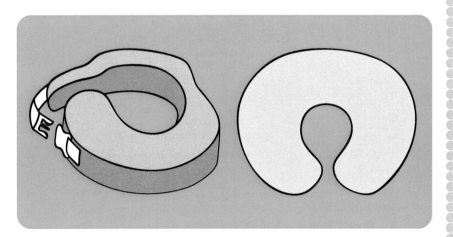

Sleepy Baby

Many babies are quite sleepy during the first few days or weeks after birth. It is important to feed your baby frequently in order for him to get enough calories as well as protect your milk supply. If your baby is still asleep and it's been three hours since the start of the last feeding, it's time to wake him up. You can do this by unwrapping his blanket and changing his diaper. Keep your baby lightly clothed or naked except for a diaper for feedings, as this will help him remain awake. Don't worry about your baby getting cold during feedings. Your body temperature will regulate to ensure that he's warm, and it is a nice opportunity for skin-to-skin contact. If your baby gets sleepy during the feeding, do some breast massage and compression to help release the milk, to remind him to suck and swallow. You can also unlatch him and lay him flat on a blanket, which wakes most newborns if they are not swaddled.

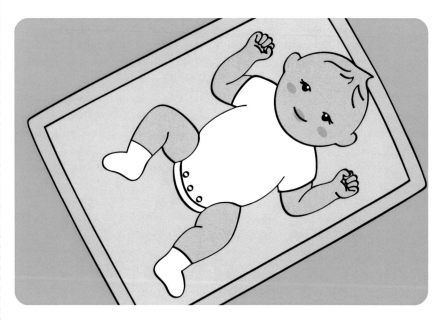

Calm Baby Before Latching

You will have a lot more success latching your baby when he is alert and calm. If your baby is crying or fussy while trying to latch, hold him upright, close to your body, and make repeated shushing sounds while gently rocking him until he calms down. You can also let him suck on your clean finger to calm him down. Trying to latch a crying baby for longer than a few minutes will probably leave you both in tears. Also, repeated latch attempts when baby is upset may cause your baby to develop a negative association with breastfeeding. It's best to calm him down first and attempt latching again in a few minutes. Try to remain calm yourself, as baby can sense your anxiety. This is a good time to revisit breathing or other relaxation techniques you may have learned during labor preparation.

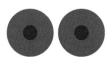

Deep Latch

If you learn only one thing from this book, it should be the importance of a deep latch. A deep latch means your baby opens his mouth wide and takes in not only your nipple but also as much of your areola as possible. Although areolas come in all sizes, the idea is for your baby to take in a mouthful of breast tissue versus just sucking on your nipple. A deep latch protects you from getting sore nipples, allows baby to transfer more milk, and protects your milk supply.

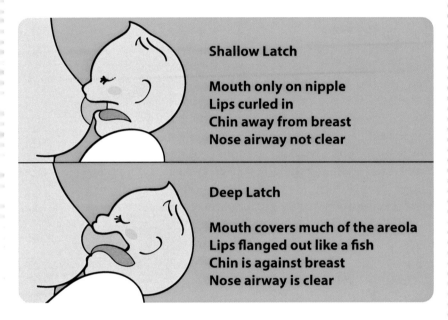

Shallow Latch

Mouth only on nipple
Lips curled in
Chin away from breast
Nose airway not clear

Deep Latch

Mouth covers much of the areola
Lips flanged out like a fish
Chin is against breast
Nose airway is clear

Breast Sandwich

The best way to achieve a deep latch is to create a breast "sandwich" with one hand to help your baby take in as much breast tissue as possible. You can create this effect by squeezing your breast to match your baby's mouth shape. Compressing your breast into a narrower shape so your baby can latch on deeply is similar to what adults do when biting into a sandwich. We hold the sandwich horizontally to match our mouth shape so that we can get a big bite. Using the cross-cradle hold, compress the underside of your breast, making a U shape with your hand, which will match your baby's vertical mouth shape. Using the football hold, compress the inside of your breast, making a C shape with your hand, which will match your baby's horizontal mouth shape in this position. Once your baby's mouth gets a little bigger, you will no longer need to shape your breast for him to latch on deeply. (See next page for illustration.)

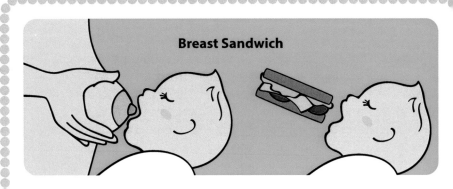

Breast Sandwich

Trouble Latching

It can be extremely frustrating when you desire to breastfeed your baby and he is not latching well or not at all. Remember that just because your baby isn't ready to latch initially doesn't mean he will *never* latch. Most babies will latch eventually. Working with a lactation consultant can be helpful when your baby is having trouble latching. In the meantime, spend lots of time holding him skin to skin. If your baby is not latching regularly and/or if you are offering any supplement, it is extremely important to protect your milk supply by pumping both breasts every three hours for fifteen minutes using a hospital-grade double electric breast pump.

Surprise Latch

I'll never forget the time I got an email from a mom I had helped previously. Her baby was now three months old and still not latching, so she was exclusively pumping and bottle feeding. One day she was just about to pump and had taken her shirt off. While holding her baby and waiting for her husband to warm a bottle, she decided to try latching her baby onto her breast. To her surprise, it worked! From then on, she was able to breastfeed regularly. Clearly, her baby was now ready.

Breastfeeding Positions

Proper positioning and latch are essential to both mom's and baby's comfort during breastfeeding. You will quickly figure out what hold works best for you and your baby with all the practice you'll be getting-and it does take practice. Some moms find that one hold works best on one breast while a different hold works best on the other breast. This may be due to your baby's preference of lying on a particular side based on his position in utero.

Cross-Cradle Hold

Cross-cradle is the most common hold moms use when learning to breastfeed a newborn after a vaginal birth. It's called "cross-cradle" because you hold your baby across your body with the opposite arm. For example, if you are feeding him on the left breast, you will support him with your right arm.

- Position the breastfeeding pillow with the widest section over your lap, close to your body.
- Place your baby on his side, with his body tucked closely into yours.
- Align baby's nose with your nipple.
- Hold baby close with your arm along the length of his body.
- Place your hand on the back of baby's neck, with your thumb and forefingers below his ears. Be sure not to cup baby's head with your hand.
- With your other hand in a U shape, hold and squeeze the underside of your breast (make a "breast sandwich").
- Make sure your fingers are not touching your areola.
- Use your nipple to stroke baby's top lip from nose to chin quickly.
- When baby opens wide, quickly bring him forward and onto your breast.
- Release the squeeze but continue holding onto your breast.

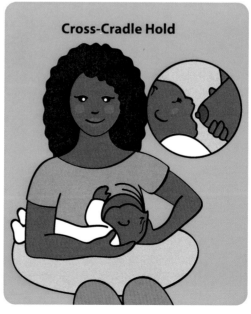

Cross-Cradle Hold

Football Hold

The football hold is an effective position to use when breastfeeding a newborn, especially after a cesarean birth, when mom is petite or baby is particularly small, when mom has large breasts, or when feeding multiples at the same time (tandem nursing).

- Lay the center of the breastfeeding pillow along the side of your body.
- Place your baby on his side on the pillow, with his body tucked closely into yours.
- Align baby's nose with your nipple.
- Hold baby close with your arm along the length of his body.
- Place your hand on the back of baby's neck, with your thumb and forefingers below his ears. Be sure not to cup baby's head with your hand.
- With your other hand in a C shape, hold and squeeze the inside of your breast (make a "breast sandwich").
- Make sure your fingers are not touching your areola.
- Use your nipple to stroke baby's top lip from nose to chin.
- When baby opens wide, quickly bring him toward you and onto your breast.
- Release the squeeze but continue holding onto your breast.

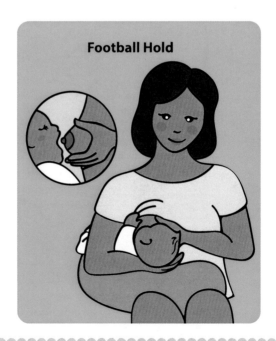

Football Hold

Cradle Hold

The cradle hold is for older babies who have more neck control. When attempting the cradle hold for the first time, start by latching baby onto your breast using the cross-cradle hold described on Page 25. Wait a few minutes until baby gets into a rhythmic sucking pattern. Then slowly release your hand from the breast you are feeding on and tuck it under baby's body, freeing up your other hand. If your baby unlatches when you attempt this, he may not have the neck control required to maintain a deep latch without you supporting his head and your breast. You can try again in a couple of weeks. Eventually, you'll be able to latch baby by bringing him toward your breast with his head supported in the crook of your elbow; you won't need to start with the cross-cradle hold.

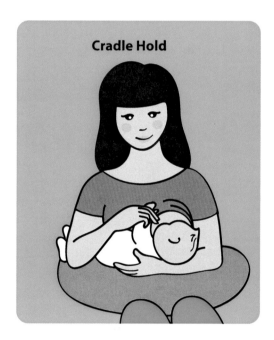

Cradle Hold

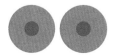

Side-Lying Position

Side-lying breastfeeding is a wonderful way to feed your baby while getting some much-needed rest. However, it can be difficult for newborn babies to obtain a deep latch in this position due to their lack of neck control. This position is best for self-latching babies after about four to six weeks.

- Lie on your side facing your baby.
- Position your baby on his side.
- Hold baby close with your arm on his back.
- Align baby's nose with your nipple and pull him in close to your body.
- With your hand in a C-shape, hold and squeeze your breast (make a "breast sandwich").
- Use your nipple to stroke baby's top lip to get him to open wide.
- Pull baby toward your breast using your arm along his back.

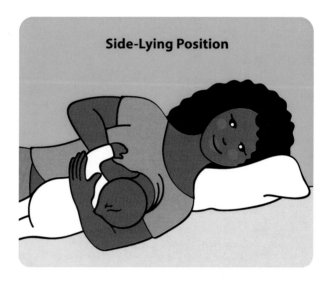

Side-Lying Position

Laid-Back Position

Laid-back breastfeeding, sometimes called biological nurturing, is a position that encourages mom and baby to use their natural instincts and reflexes to breastfeed comfortably and successfully without any rigid rules or instructions for positioning and latch. This position leaves moms hands free while baby breastfeeds. It's a good position for mom's who have an overactive letdown, as it works against gravity to slow the milk flow. You don't need to do much to get baby latched onto the breast in this position. Just support baby's body and let his natural instincts lead him.

- Lie back comfortably in a chair or bed while holding baby upright facing your bare chest.
- Lower baby so his nose aligns with your nipple.
- When ready, baby will start lifting his head, searching for the breast.
- Baby will lift his head, open his mouth, and latch onto the breast.
- If the latch doesn't seem right to him, he will unlatch and try again.
- If the latch feels uncomfortable to you, unlatch him and let him try again.

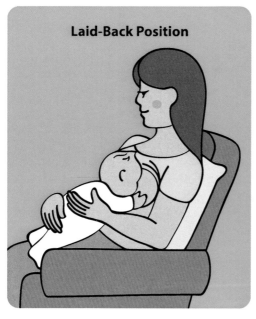

Laid-Back Position

Breastfeeding Multiples

In the first few weeks after your twins or multiples arrive, it's best to work with each baby on their own as they learn to latch on and transfer milk. Once breastfeeding is established and the babies are latching correctly, you can feed two babies at once (tandem feeding), making feedings more efficient. Breastfeeding pillows made for feeding twins can be helpful, as can reaching out for support to a lactation consultant or a parents-of-multiples group.

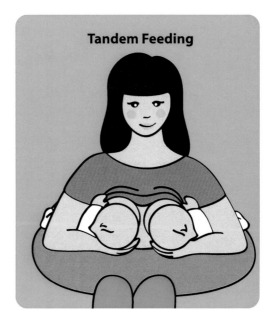

Tandem Feeding

Unlatching

To unlatch your baby from your breast in any position, place your finger at the corner of baby's mouth and pull baby's skin away from the breast to break the seal. Another option is to slide your clean index finger inside your baby's mouth on one side, between his gums, and gently twist your finger until he releases the breast.

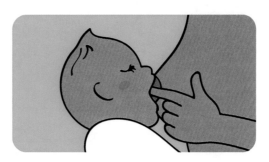

Ideally, mom's nipple should be perfectly round when baby comes off the breast after a feeding. If baby was not latched deeply enough, your nipple may look compressed and pointed, like a new tube of lipstick. If this happens, continue to work on obtaining a deep latch and seek the help of a lactation consultant if necessary.

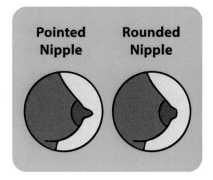

Pointed Nipple **Rounded Nipple**

Burping

It's always a good idea to attempt to burp your baby after each breast during a feeding session. Because your baby will ingest a relatively low volume of milk during the first few days, he may not produce a burp. There's no need to spend a long time trying to get your baby to burp. Simply try for a few minutes after each breast. Most parents of newborns feel comfortable using one of two burping positions. The first is to simply bring your baby onto your upper chest, allowing his upper body to rest on your shoulder. Gently pat and/or rub his back to encourage him to burp. The second position is to sit your baby on your lap facing sideways. Keep one of your hands behind his back at all times in case he leans back. Place your other hand along your baby's jawline, letting him rest his jaw on your hand. Your hand should not touch his neck, only his jawline. Gently pat and/or rub his back, encouraging him to burp. During a feeding, if your baby frequently unlatches for no apparent reason, he may need to stop to burp before continuing.

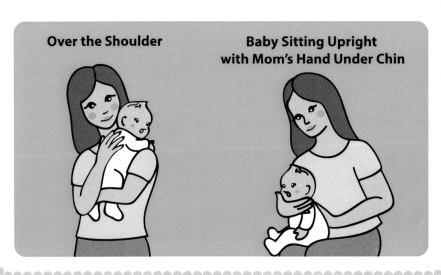

Over the Shoulder **Baby Sitting Upright with Mom's Hand Under Chin**

CHAPTER 4
WHEN AND HOW OFTEN TO FEED BABY

As a new parent, you may be wondering how to tell when your baby is hungry and how often to feed her. She will eat quite frequently in the early weeks as she learns to breastfeed and as your milk supply increases. Before you know it, you will become an expert on reading your baby's hunger cues.

Frequent Feedings

You might be surprised to learn that it's completely normal for your newborn to breastfeed 8 to 12 times or more in a 24-hour period. You may feel like all you are doing is breastfeeding! If you can, think about these early weeks of frequent feeding as a time to bond with your baby and build your milk supply. Once breastfeeding is established and comfortable, feeding sessions can actually be a nice respite when you and your baby can spend some quiet downtime together.

You'll want to feed your newborn on demand (whenever she shows signs of hunger) and at least every three hours from the start of one feeding till the start of the next, around the clock. Once your baby regains her birth weight, ideally by two weeks of age, most pediatricians and lactation consultants are comfortable letting her wake up on her own for nighttime feedings instead of having you wake her every three hours.

Newborn Tummy Size

On day one of your baby's life, her tummy is the size of a cherry and can hold only about one teaspoon of milk. Because she can't store more milk, she will need to eat frequently. Her tummy size will increase quickly, allowing her to take in more milk per feeding, which may extend the time between feedings.

Newborn Tummy Size				
Age of Baby	One Day	Three Days	One Week	One Month
Capacity	1 tsp.	0.75-1 oz.	1.5-2 oz.	2.5-4 oz.

Demand and Supply

As your baby sucks and removes milk from your breasts (demand), she is programming your body with instructions on how much milk to continue making (supply). If your baby typically removes about two ounces of milk per feeding, that tells your body to continue making at least two ounces of milk for future feedings. The greater her demand for milk, the greater your milk supply will be. The first six weeks is a critical time for establishing your milk supply, so continue feeding on demand and reap the rewards of a healthy milk supply going forward. During that time, it is important not to drastically change the frequency of feedings. If your baby won't latch on to one of your breasts or your nipples are too sore to breastfeed, you'll need to use a breast pump every three hours to protect your milk supply. Any changes to the frequency of feedings should be gradual to avoid developing a breast infection.

Hunger Signs

Because babies cannot talk, they show us what they need with their bodies. Early signs of hunger can be as subtle as your baby moving her lips or tongue. She then will begin to make larger movements, such as putting her hand to her mouth, and will display the rooting reflex, turning her head toward her caregiver's chest when held, as if she is trying to latch on. Babies will do this even with dad or another caregiver who is unable to breastfeed! If she is still not fed, she will get upset and cry. It's always best to catch one of the early hunger signs and feed baby before she gets too upset to breastfeed. If you missed the early hunger signs and baby is extremely upset, try to calm her before attempting to latch by holding and rocking her or offering her your clean finger to suck on.

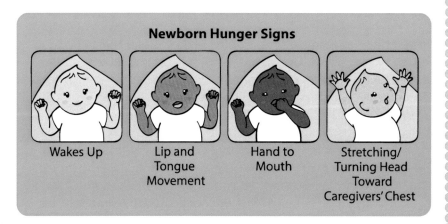

Newborn Hunger Signs

Wakes Up | Lip and Tongue Movement | Hand to Mouth | Stretching/Turning Head Toward Caregivers' Chest

Routine vs. Schedule

I do not recommend putting your baby on a strict breastfeeding schedule. Your baby may be hungrier at particular times of day or may not have taken in much milk at the last feeding. Look at your baby instead of looking at the clock. If she displays hunger signs, you can assume she is hungry. I recommend a feeding routine rather than a schedule. Most babies like predictability and enjoy the routine of sleep-eat-play. Since newborns sleep so frequently, I recommend feeding them as soon as they wake up. Every baby is different, but eventually most babies will put themselves on a schedule. Having said that, I *do* recommend feeding your baby at least every three hours from the start of one feeding to the start of the next feeding during the day-and more often if she shows hunger signs. This will help encourage your baby to feed more frequently during the day and eventually sleep for a longer stretch at night.

Cluster Feedings

Frequent or cluster feedings are common and normal in the first few weeks of life. Your baby is still learning how to take in a greater volume of milk at longer intervals. As she grows and becomes stronger, she will become more efficient at breastfeeding, leading to shorter and less frequent feedings. Most babies take in more milk in the middle of the night and the early morning hours when prolactin, the hormone that makes milk, is at its highest. Milk supply is typically lower in the evening hours, which often leads to frequent feedings. Babies also cluster feed during growth spurts, which commonly occur at around two to three weeks, six weeks, twelve weeks, three months, six months and nine months.

Milk Composition

Breastmilk contains everything your baby needs for the first four to six months of life, including proteins, fats, carbohydrates, vitamins and minerals, enzymes, hormones, and immune system protectors. Some moms wonder if they will continue to have enough milk for their growing baby. Amazingly, the composition of your breastmilk will change automatically over time to meet your baby's developing needs. When your baby reaches about ten pounds, the amount of milk she takes in per feeding will remain approximately the same for the remainder of your breastfeeding experience. At this point, babies typically take about three or four ounces per feeding for a total of about 24 to 36 ounces per day (an average of about 1 to 1.5 ounces per hour). Even as your baby begins to take solids, your breastmilk will continue to be a main source of nutrition throughout her first year of life.

Weight Loss and Weight Gain

It is normal for newborns to lose up to ten percent of their birth weight in the first four days of life. Babies usually start gaining weight on day five. If your baby has lost ten percent or more of her birth weight, seek the help of a lactation consultant to ensure that she is getting enough milk. Lactation consultants and pediatricians typically want babies to regain their birth weight by two weeks of age or sooner. It is perfectly normal to be concerned about whether your baby is getting enough milk. If you are breastfeeding frequently and your health care provider is not concerned about her weight, you can assume she is getting enough.

Average Weight Gain	
Days 1 - 4	Weight loss of up to 10% is considered normal
Day 5 thru 5 months	Weight gain of about 5 - 7 ounces per week
By 2 weeks	Baby should have regained birth weight
By 5 - 6 months	Baby should have doubled birth weight
6 - 12 months	Weight gain of about 3 - 5 ounces per week
By 12 months	Baby should have tripled birth weight

Is Baby Drinking?

Sometimes it's hard to tell if your baby is actually transferring milk or if she is just sucking for comfort at the breast. Look for active jaw movement from her chin all the way up to her ear. You can also look for a pause in the sucking pattern when baby's mouth is open at its widest, indicating a swallow. The longer the pause, the greater the amount of milk baby is swallowing. If baby is indeed drinking, your breasts will feel softer and less full after feedings. Also, baby will seem satiated and will no longer show signs of hunger.

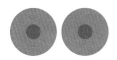

Is Baby Finished?

It can be difficult to tell when baby has had enough milk when breastfeeding. The amount of active sucking time during a breastfeeding session can range from 10 to 45 minutes total from both breasts, depending on mom's milk supply and baby's efficiency. Therefore, it's best to watch your baby instead of the clock. When sucking slows from an active suck to a more pacifying suck, if she falls asleep after at least ten minutes of active sucking, or she comes off the breast, she is probably done on that side. Try to burp her and then offer the second breast. Your baby may not nurse from both breasts at every feeding session, but it's a good idea to offer both sides in order to protect your milk supply. Don't worry about trying to "drain your breasts." Your breasts are never really empty because as soon as milk is removed, more milk is produced. Some moms worry about a foremilk/hindmilk imbalance. Foremilk is the initial, watery milk baby gets while breastfeeding. As she stays on the breast, the milk becomes thicker and higher in fat, called the hindmilk. Allowing your baby to suck for as long as the sucking is active on both sides should ensure she is getting enough of both foremilk and hindmilk.

Is Baby Getting Enough?

You can feel confident that your baby is getting enough milk if:

- Milk volume increases by day four.
- Wet diapers increase by day five.
- Baby's poop is yellow by day five.
- Baby has an appropriate number of pees and poops per day.
- Baby is eating at least eight times in a 24-hour period.
- Baby is actively sucking for 10 to 45 minutes per feeding.
- Breasts feel softer after feedings.
- Baby seems content after feedings.
- Baby is gaining an appropriate amount of weight.

If your suspect that your baby is not getting enough milk, contact your pediatrician and/or lactation consultant as soon as possible.

Pee and Poop

Lactation consultants often ask about baby's pee and poop because the color, consistency, and frequency tell us a lot about how breastfeeding is going. The amount of pee and poop baby is expelling tells us how much milk baby is ingesting. Breastmilk poop after day four should appear yellow in color and may be somewhat seedy in texture. Some say it looks like mustard mixed with cottage cheese. Don't be alarmed if your baby's poop appears to be very loose. Until your baby begins eating solids, the consistency of her poop will reflect her liquid diet. If you are supplementing with any amount of formula, your baby's poop may be thicker and more brown in color. She will probably poop less frequently, since it takes longer for baby's digestive system to break down formula.

Pee and Poop Guidelines					
	Day 1	Day 2	Day 3	Day 4	Day 5 +
Number of Pees	1+	2+	3+	4+	6+
Number of Poops	1-2	1-2	1-3	0-3	3-6+
Color of Poop	Black	Black/ Green	Brown/ Green	Brown/ Green/ Yellow	Yellow/ Seedy/ Soft

It may seem odd that baby may not poop at all on day 4 in the table above. During the first three days, baby's poop is a product of the amniotic fluid she drank while in the womb. On day 4 or 5, baby's poop becomes a product of the colostrum she is getting from mom's breast. Therefore, there may be a temporary pause on day four while mom's milk supply increases. As your baby grows, the number of bowel movements per day will significantly decrease. By about 4 to 6 weeks of age, she may poop as little as once per day or even once per week! This is completely normal. Look for a weight gain of 1 to 2 pounds per month and at least five wet diapers per day.

Input and Output

I remember working with a family who just had their first baby. Mom was busy breastfeeding frequently and her husband was trying to help out in other ways. After the baby was breastfed, her husband brought the baby to the nursery for a diaper change. As soon as he brought the baby back into the family room, the baby pooped again. The dad told the mom that it was her turn to change baby's diaper. Mom said, "No way, I'm in charge of input and you're in charge of output!"

Shorter Feedings

As your baby grows bigger and stronger, she will become more and more efficient at the breast. She will be able to take in more milk during feedings in a shorter amount of time. Therefore, don't be surprised if your baby's feeding sessions become shorter and/or if she can now go longer between feedings. It's still a good idea to aim for feeding your baby at least every three hours from start to start of daytime feedings to encourage her to sleep longer at night and to protect your milk supply.

Dessert Trick

After breastfeeding, your baby will often be peacefully asleep in your arms. However, she may need a diaper change or even a change of clothes after a feeding. Following all of this activity, your baby likely will be wide awake again and it can take time to settle her back to sleep. In these cases, I like to recommend the dessert trick. Once you change and swaddle your baby, put her back onto the breast she last fed on to give her a little dessert. Within five minutes, your baby will most likely be asleep again. But don't rush to return her to her crib or bassinet. Wait about 15 to 20 minutes until your baby is in a deep sleep so she won't wake up again when you put her down.

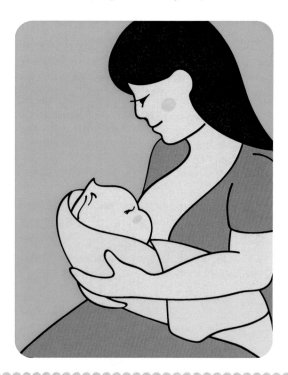

CHAPTER 5
LIFE WITH A NEWBORN

The first few weeks with your newborn will likely be filled with joy as you cherish your baby's long-anticipated arrival. At the same time, you may feel overwhelmed by your new role: taking care of a tiny human being. No matter how much warning you receive about the lack of sleep or lifestyle changes that accompany your baby's arrival, nothing can truly prepare you for what life is like with a newborn. As one pediatrician I know put it, "it's not hard, it's just… constant." Caring for a newborn truly is a 24-hour-a-day job. You'll need all the support you can get.

Adjusting to Motherhood

One major change that occurs once you become a mother is that you will no longer be able to do whatever you want, whenever you want. It's amazing how one tiny baby can affect your best-laid plans. Between frequent feedings, diapering, burping, swaddling, and soothing your baby to sleep, you will be busy nearly every waking moment. You may still be healing from the birth and may experience some pain with breastfeeding. You may feel moody and emotional for no reason or may not feel like yourself. This is all completely normal-your shifting hormones are to blame. So rest whenever you can and make caring for your newborn your main priority. Accept any help or food that is offered. You will never appreciate a home-cooked meal delivered to you as much as you will during this time.

The Fourth Trimester

The first three months after the birth of your baby are often referred to as the fourth trimester. Although babies are born after nine months of gestation, newborns are physiologically more suited to the environment they experienced in the womb, where it was dark, warm, and cozy. Inside, your baby heard constant white noise while being gently lulled to sleep by your movement. The world outside the womb is bright, loud, and sometimes cold, especially when baby is away from a caregiver's arms. To help your newborn feel as comfortable and calm as possible, try to recreate a womb-like environment. When baby was inside you, he was constantly held and rocked. When baby is fussy or when you are trying to help him sleep, you can rock him, swing him, or simply walk around with him. Wearing your baby in a front carrier, wrap, or sling-where he can feel your warmth, smell your scent, and hear your heartbeat-also will comfort him. Another way to recreate a womb-like experience is to use a swaddle or a sleep sack to wrap your baby for sleep. He had little room to stretch out in the womb and his crib will feel enormous to him. The swaddle will prevent his involuntary arm movements from waking him up. Lastly, using a white noise machine will help calm him and will mask any sudden environmental noise if he's a light sleeper.

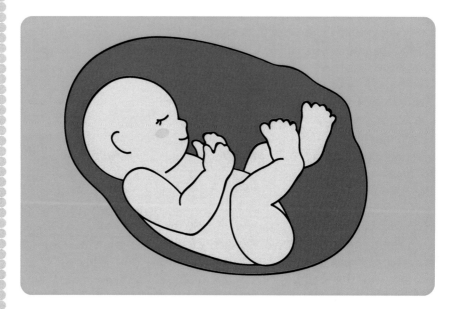

Are you wearing her?

I'll never forget when my older sister, already a mom, came to visit when my first baby was two weeks old. I complained that I didn't know how to comfort my daughter when she cried. "Are you wearing her when she gets fussy?" my sister asked. Umm, no... That day she took me to purchase a front carrier and what a difference that made. My daughter would snuggle up next to me in her carrier and often fall asleep as I held and comforted her. I wish I had known what she needed, right from the start.

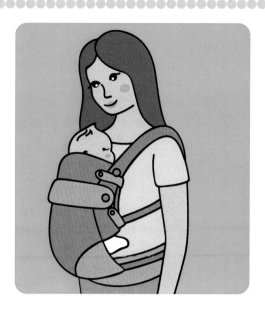

Newborn Sleep

Newborns sleep approximately 16 to 20 hours per day and are awake only for feedings, diaper changes, and short periods of alertness before they are ready to sleep again. If your baby gets fussy after being awake for about an hour, this usually means he is ready to go back to sleep. Despite the term "sleep like a baby," most newborns need help getting to sleep. Once he falls asleep, it takes about 15 to 20 minutes for your baby to enter a deep sleep cycle that will allow you to lay him down successfully without him waking up. Newborns also often have their days and nights mixed up. When you were pregnant, your active daytime movement lulled your baby to sleep. At night, your baby probably was more alert, when you weren't! To reverse this pattern, try to feed your baby at least every three hours-or even more frequently-during the day. A baby who sleeps between 6 to 8 hours at night is considered to be "sleeping through the night." This doesn't typically happen before baby is three months of age or weighs at least twelve pounds. Many babies do not consistently sleep through the night until closer to their first birthday or even later. As your baby begins to sleep longer, your milk supply will automatically adjust to the new demand. If you are struggling with engorgement during this transition, see "Treating Engorgement" on page 55.

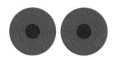

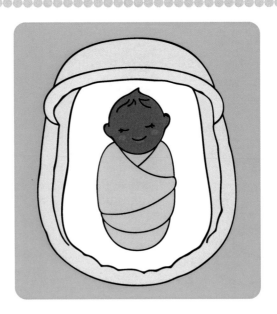

Deep Sleep

One couple I saw was confused about why baby's grandma was always successful putting their baby down to sleep, but when the parents tried to put her down, she would wake up and start crying within five minutes. It turned out that grandma was enjoying holding the baby so much that she didn't want to put her down as soon as she fell asleep. I explained that once grandma finally did put their baby down after at least 15 to 20 minutes of holding, she was in a deep enough sleep that she didn't wake up when grandma laid her down.

Sleep Deprivation

There's no doubt that the first few months of your newborn's life will lead to sleep deprivation for you. Frequent feedings will cause you to wake at least every three hours. However, rest is crucial for healing and your milk supply. So, during the early weeks, you will need to prioritize sleeping over other activities... like answering email, checking in at work, or keeping your house sparkling clean. Some people recommend sleeping when the baby sleeps. This is ideal if you have helpers to take care of meal prep, laundry, and cleaning. Try to rest when baby naps, even if you don't actually sleep. When you sleep-even for 20 or 30 minutes-your body produces prolactin, the hormone that works to increase your milk supply. You'll hopefully feel refreshed and better able to cope with whatever the rest of your day brings. Getting outside at least once every day for fresh air can help you feel less tired, too.

Crying and Fussiness

One of the hardest things to do as a parent is to listen to your baby cry. Crying triggers an emotional response so strong that you'll want to do whatever is necessary to stop it as soon as possible. Remember that a baby's cry is meant to be uncomfortable for parents. This discomfort ensures that babies get their needs met. Crying is your baby's only way to communicate out loud at this point in his young life. He is rarely as desperate as his cry would make you think. Because your baby will pick up on your anxiety, try to remain calm as you attempt to figure out what he needs. If you can't determine what baby needs, try holding him close in a dark, quiet room. He may simply be overstimulated and want some quiet time with mom.

Fussy Baby Checklist

One mom I know posted a checklist on her fridge that she went through every time her baby was fussy. The list included things like: needs diaper change, hungry, too hot, too cold, gassy, tired, and wants to be held. She was usually able to figure out why her baby was fussy by the time she got to the end of the list. Sometimes, something as simple as a change in environment, like taking a walk around the block, works to calm a newborn.

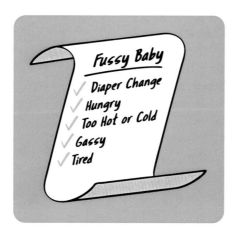

Baby Wearing

One of the best ways to calm a fussy baby is to wear him in a front carrier, wrap, or sling. Your baby may be having trouble adjusting to his new world and having you wear him is the next best thing to being back inside of you. He will be comforted by the close proximity to you, hearing your heart beat, and smelling your exclusive scent, a similar experience to when he is held skin to skin. He will most likely drift off to sleep while being

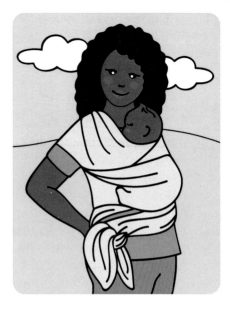

held. Although most babies enjoy being worn this way, it is important for his development to give him plenty of opportunities to stretch out his arms, legs, and neck. You can do this during the short period of awake times after feedings, lying on a blanket, and/or under a baby gym.

Playing with Your Newborn

Most newborns cannot stay awake for more than about an hour at a time and are usually ready to sleep shortly after feedings. If your baby does not seem sleepy right after a feeding, it's time to play! Playtime

with your newborn may simply mean holding him and talking or singing to him. He will love looking at your face and may try to mimic your movements, like sticking out his tongue when you stick out yours. Newborns can see only about eight to twelve inches away and don't see color until about five months of age. They tend to focus on high-contrast items, since that's what they see best with their initial blurry vision. You can print out or purchase

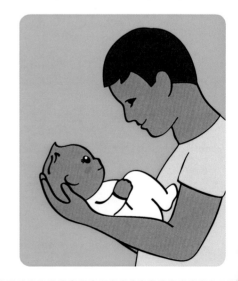

high-contrast black and white images to place next to your baby when he is awake. Babies are like little sponges at this point, so having something to look at will promote his brain development. The duration of awake/alert time after feedings is usually quite short, often only five or ten minutes. When baby starts yawning, stops making eye contact, or gets fussy after being awake for about an hour, he is probably ready to go back to sleep.

Tummy Time

Starting in 1994, parents were encouraged to put babies to sleep on their backs to reduce the risk of SIDS (Sudden Infant Death Syndrome). This recommendation has significantly reduced the occurrence of SIDS. However, because babies spend so much time on their backs, many aren't spending enough time on their tummies. Tummy time is important for baby's neck, mouth, tongue, and upper body development. It also helps to prevent baby's head from becoming flat in one area from lying on the same spot. Try to have your baby spend some time on his tummy while he's awake at least twice a day, even for a few minutes at a time, to help him get used to the feeling. You can also accomplish this by holding him on your chest while you are lying down and letting him lift his head to look at you. A good way to remember to do tummy time is to do it consistently after daytime feedings. You may want to roll up a blanket or towel and place it under your baby's chest to provide room for him to move his head from side to side. For more information on tummy time, visit www.tummytimemethod.com.

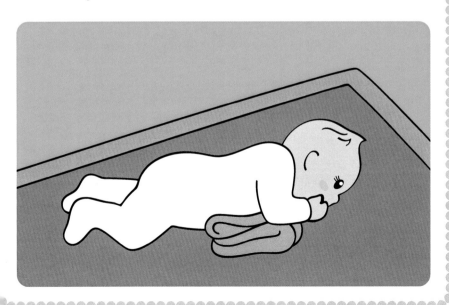

Older Siblings

Older siblings are often excited about the new baby's arrival. Making a big deal out of becoming a big sister or big brother lets them know that, although there's a new baby around, they are still an important part of the family. If they are old enough, ask for their help getting a diaper or burp cloth for you. This will help them to feel good about themselves as they contribute to the family's well-being. If your older child feels jealous or frustrated with all the time you spend breastfeeding your newborn, put together a basket of new or special toys and books that your older child can play with only while you are breastfeeding. This is also a wonderful time for your older child to develop a strong bond with dad, partner, or grandparents.

Partner Support

During these first few weeks, you will spend an extraordinary number of hours caring for your newborn. It will be an extremely busy time and teamwork is essential. Although your partner will not be able to help with breastfeeding directly, there are many other things your partner can do to support your breastfeeding journey, especially in the beginning. Your partner can bring you water and snacks while you are breastfeeding. They can also support you simply by offering encouragement, telling you what an important and terrific job you are doing, and reminding you of your breastfeeding goals when you feel tired or frustrated. They can also reach out to find lactation support if necessary.

Your partner can bond with the baby by doing the burping, diaper changing, and soothing to sleep. It will be important for your partner to figure out the best ways to care for and soothe the baby, which may be different from how you do things. Encourage this bonding time and enjoy a much-needed break for yourself. If possible, try to take a daily walk together to get some fresh air and to nurture your adult relationship. There will be constant distractions but try to continue to make time for each other. Taking a few minutes to reconnect each day can make a big difference.

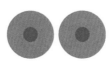

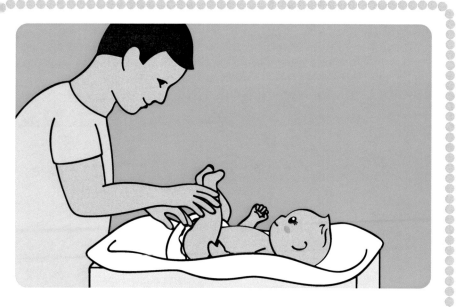

Peanut Butter and Jelly

One mom shared with me that her husband made her a peanut butter and jelly sandwich every night before he went to bed. He would wrap it up on a plate and leave it on the table next to where she would be breastfeeding during the night. Sometimes she ate it and sometimes she didn't, but this simple act of kindness showed her that he supported and appreciated what she was doing for their baby. I thought this was so touching.

Visitors

Friends and family will likely want to meet your new baby as soon as possible. Accept visitors only when you feel ready and only as often as you feel comfortable. Don't be shy about asking them for help with the baby, an older sibling, or household tasks. They are more rested than you are and most want to help however they can. If you're lucky, visitors will bring a snack to enjoy together or a meal for later. Holding and rocking your baby to sleep after a feeding is a perfect job for visiting helpers. You will love the time to yourself to go to the bathroom, shower, or eat, and they will love having snuggle time with baby. Friends who have experience with breastfeeding can be an invaluable resource and most enjoy sharing their stories and offering advice and support. If you feel overwhelmed by frequent visits, keep them short and sweet. If you anticipate that any visitors will be unsupportive of breastfeeding or add stress to your household, interfering with this special bonding time, it's best to wait until you feel healed, rested, and emotionally strong before inviting them to visit.

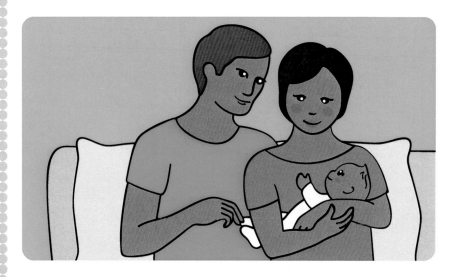

Postpartum Doula or Night Nurse

If you do not have family available or feel like you need some extra help, you may want to hire a postpartum doula or night nurse. Postpartum doulas are available during the day and evenings and sometimes overnight. They provide tremendous support and education about caring for your new baby. Some have also been trained to assist with breastfeeding. Night nurses or night doulas help by bringing baby to you for feedings and then taking care of the diapering, burping, and soothing baby back to sleep. Although these resources can be costly, they can be an enormous help when necessary, even if only for a short period of time. For more information or to find a doula in your area, visit DONA (www.dona.org).

Getting Out of the House

Most moms in our modern world end up spending much of their time alone inside their homes with their babies. Although it's easier to stay home with a newborn, try to get out of the house with your baby at least once a day. Remaining home may become overwhelming and isolating and you may not realize how you feel until you leave the house. It's healthier to get out and interact with others as you learn to manage your new role as a parent. Taking a walk with baby or doing light exercise, either alone or with a group of other moms, can be supportive and healthy for both of you.

Breastfeeding in Public

Once you get the hang of breastfeeding, you will start to feel ready to leave the house and breastfeed in public. Breastfeeding while you are out and about is convenient-no bottles to carry and no worrying about where to warm them up. Many moms like to use a nursing cover or blanket to cover their breasts while breastfeeding in public, although this is not necessary. You have the right to feed your baby wherever you have the right to be. If you are planning your first outing, a breastfeeding support group is a great place to nurse in public in a welcoming environment.

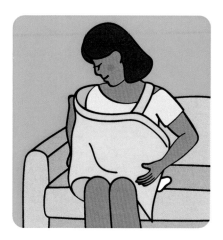

Wearing a nursing bra or tank top and a nursing shirt make accessing the breasts for feedings much easier, whether you are home or out and about. There's a large market for these types of clothes and you should be able to find comfortable nursing wear either in stores or online.

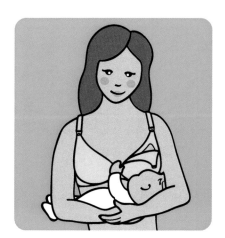
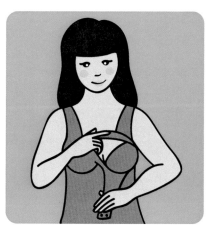

It's Just a Boob

I'll never forget the first time my friend and I nursed our newborns in public. We were sitting at a little café encouraging each other to go ahead and breastfeed. Although we both felt nervous, we kept saying "It's just a boob." This got us laughing so hard that we forgot how nervous we were. Suddenly, we both felt comfortable enough to breastfeed at that café, and many other places after that. It was so liberating to be able to take our babies anywhere we wanted to go without the inconvenience of carrying bottles.

Breastfeeding Support Groups

Many hospitals and parenting centers offer weekly breastfeeding support groups for new moms. These groups are a place to get your questions answered, learn from other people's questions and experiences, meet new friends, and observe others breastfeeding in a supportive environment. If your local hospital does not offer a breastfeeding support group, visit the La Leche League International website to find a local group (www.llli.org/get-help/).

Mothers'/Parents' Clubs

Mothers' and/or parents' clubs provide a way to meet other young families in your area who have similarly aged babies. They usually meet weekly, often at a member's home, and many clubs host regular events, such as family outings and speakers. These groups typically offer an online forum where you can ask questions of other members regarding parenting issues or seek recommendations for a babysitter, preschool, or even a plumber or contractor. As your little one grows, your playgroup may move meet-ups to a park, so the toddlers can play outside while the parents socialize. This time with other moms is so important, especially for new moms, as it helps to reduce anxiety about parenting and prevent feelings of postpartum depression due to social isolation. Your baby will benefit too, learning social skills such as sharing and empathy through play. Moms provide such a strong support network for one another and these relationships often last a lifetime.

Postpartum Depression

Becoming a parent is a life-changing event that can feel overwhelming. Hormonal shifts during the postpartum period can often bring on the baby blues, a normal phase that should pass quickly. Unfortunately, postpartum mood disorders such as depression and anxiety are increasingly common. Between 50 and 85 percent of new moms experience some level of depression during the postpartum period. If your symptoms persist or become debilitating, or you are at all concerned about your mental health or the safety of yourself or your baby, don't be shy about seeking professional help. There are numerous therapists and psychologists who specialize in helping postpartum moms. Postpartum Support International provides resources and local referrals (www.postpartum.net). There are also medications for anxiety and depression that are safe to take while breastfeeding.

Some signs and symptoms of postpartum depression are:

- Feeling sad and hopeless with frequent crying
- Feeling anxious, irritable or restless
- Oversleeping or insomnia
- Trouble concentrating
- Losing interest in activities
- Overeating or not eating enough
- Avoiding friends and family
- Difficulty bonding with baby
- Feeling unable to care for baby
- Thinking about harming self or baby

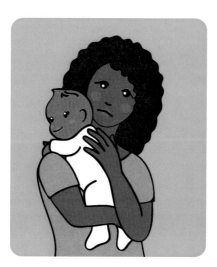

CHAPTER 6
COMMON CHALLENGES

Although many women go on to meet or exceed their breastfeeding goals, the road to comfortable breastfeeding may be a little rocky as you learn this new skill. However, you can overcome most common challenges by educating yourself ahead of time and having a good support system in place. If you are experiencing any of these challenges, contact a lactation consultant for assistance. The sooner the problem is alleviated, the sooner you can get back to comfortable breastfeeding. Sometimes the slightest change can make a huge difference.

Uterine Contractions

During the first week, your uterus will contract during breastfeeding as it works toward returning to its pre-pregnancy size. This can cause abdominal pain while breastfeeding. The pain should last only a few days but can be uncomfortable. If necessary, ask your obstetrician about safe pain medicine to take before breastfeeding. Uterine contractions while breastfeeding may be more intense with second and subsequent babies.

Sore Nipples

One of the most common complaints from new moms is sore nipples. Breastfeeding shouldn't hurt, but that doesn't mean that your nipples won't feel a bit tender as you and your baby learn this new skill. The main cause of nipple soreness is a shallow latch, when baby is sucking only on mom's nipple instead of also taking more of the areola into her mouth. In the initial weeks, some moms experience slight discomfort when baby first latches. This pain typically subsides after about a minute or once milk begins to flow, and doesn't necessarily indicate a poor latch. Breastfeeding with continuous pain during the entire feeding can cause your nipples to blister, crack, or even bleed. Once the skin breaks down, bacteria from your baby's mouth can enter the breast tissue and may cause a breast infection. Seek help from a lactation consultant if you experience severe nipple pain, if your nipples are blistered, cracked, or bleeding, or if you are having trouble obtaining a deep latch. Note that your nipples can be damaged by only a few feedings with a shallow latch, so get help as soon as possible.

Nipple Care

Avoid using soap on your nipples as this can remove the natural oils that keep your nipples and areola lubricated. The run-off from shampooing your hair and soaping up the rest of your body will leave your breasts and nipples clean. Avoid harsh laundry detergents when washing nursing bras, as this can cause nipple dryness and can exacerbate any soreness you are experiencing.

Sore Nipple Treatment

The first step in treating sore nipples is to improve your positioning and latch. (See page 23 on obtaining a deep latch.) Some moms find it helpful to switch breastfeeding positions while healing so baby's tongue isn't compressing the same spot of the nipple at every feeding. As your baby learns to latch deeply onto your breast tissue, your nipples will begin to heal. In the meantime, topical nipple creams and oils can increase your comfort. Coconut oil works especially well to heal sore nipples. There is no need to wash these off before feeding your baby. If greasy residue on your nipple and areola prevents your baby from maintaining a deep latch, gently wipe it off with a soft cloth before latching.

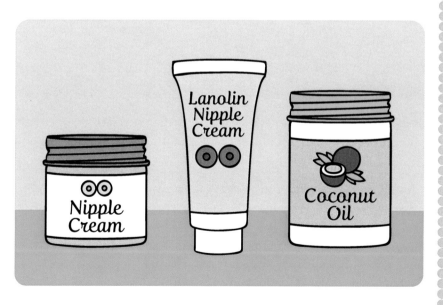

If nipple creams or oils don't provide enough relief, you may want to try using hydrogel pads, which can be more healing. These pads are a wet-wound healing method and should be worn inside your bra day and night except when feeding or showering. They feel especially nice after feedings if you store them in their packaging in the refrigerator while breastfeeding. Check the suggested usage duration on the box, as some gel pads last only 24 hours while others are good for multiple days. Do not use any creams or oils while using hydrogel pads.

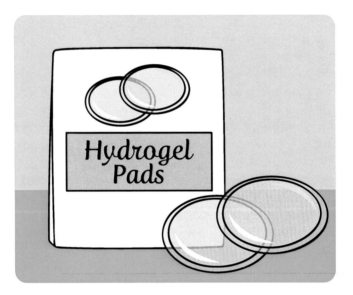

Engorgement

Engorgement is a swelling of the breast tissue caused by the increase in milk volume that typically begins sometime between days four and six. Your breasts may feel heavy, warm to the touch, and lumpy, especially on the outer sides and under your arms. Some moms suspect the lumps they feel are plugged ducts; however, plugged ducts do not typically occur before two weeks postpartum. Plugged ducts are much smaller (pea-sized) and are located closer to the areola. (See page 63 for more information.) The skin on your breasts may appear red and may also feel tight. You may develop a slight fever of 100 degrees Fahrenheit or less during this time. Postpartum engorgement typically lasts anywhere from 24 to 72 hours and is completely normal. The breasts initially create an oversupply to ensure there is enough milk for your baby. As your baby breastfeeds, she programs your body to produce as much milk as she needs per feeding. If you are feeding your baby on demand and she is removing milk regularly and efficiently, you may not feel any engorgement at all. After about two or three weeks, your breasts will no longer feel as full as they did at first. This is normal and does not mean that your milk supply has decreased. It just means that your body now knows just how much milk to make for your baby. You most likely will not feel that fullness again unless you are separated from your baby at a feeding time, your baby sleeps longer than expected between feedings, or you are in the process of weaning.

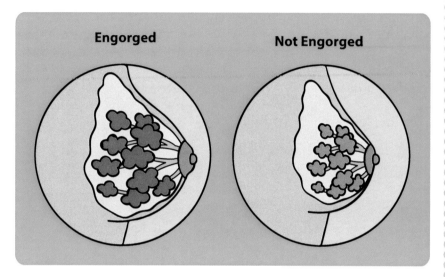

Treating Engorgement

Some ways to prevent and treat engorgement are:

- Frequent feedings (on demand, not scheduled)
- Gentle breast massage; small circular motion with fingertips before and/or during feedings
- Warm shower or warm compresses before feedings
- Cold compresses after feedings (bags of frozen vegetables covered in thin cloth work well)
- Manual expression of milk before latching, to soften the breast
- Pumping with an electric pump for no more than five minutes
- Wear a supportive bra (no underwire)
- Avoid pacifiers

Cabbage Leaves for Treating Engorgement

If you are still uncomfortably full after trying these suggested treatment methods for engorgement, you can try using green cabbage leaves. Cabbage leaves work similarly to cold compresses to reduce swelling. Keep the cabbage in the refrigerator and use after feedings. Remove two leaves and wash and dry them before use. Roll a soup can or a rolling pin over the leaves in order to break up the veins. This will help release the sulfur, which can help reduce the swelling. Cut each leaf lengthwise and place the two halves inside your bra, covering the breasts but not the nipples. Leave the cabbage leaves inside your bra for no more than twenty minutes. Repeat this process two to three times per day and discontinue use as soon as you feel more comfortable. Please note that prolonged use of cabbage leaves inside your bra can lead to significantly reduced milk supply.

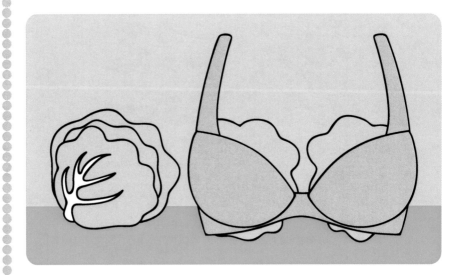

Leaking

Some moms experience leaking of breastmilk during the first few weeks as their bodies get the message about how much milk their babies need. You may leak from one side while breastfeeding on the other side, or from both breasts in between feedings. Nursing pads work well to catch excess milk. Be sure to change pads whenever they become moist to avoid an overgrowth of yeast on your breasts, which can lead to thrush, (See page 62.) You can purchase reusable cloth pads, which you'll need to wash between uses, or disposable pads, which are convenient for frequent leaking. In addition to breast pads, there are products on the market that you wear inside your bra to collect excess milk between or during feedings, or even while you're sleeping. (Milkies: www.mymilkies.com.) Another option is a silicone breast pump, which uses suction to attach to your breast, collecting milk from one side while you feed on the other. (Haakaa Silicon Breast Pump: www.haakaausa.com.) These products are good options for moms who experience excessive leaking and who want to save milk for future feedings.

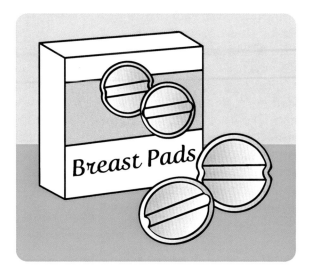

Spit-Up

Spitting up after feedings is common because your baby's digestive system is immature. The apparent volume of spit-up often concerns parents, who wonder if baby just spit-up her entire meal. Keep in mind that the volume often appears greater than it is, and babies aren't usually hungry right after spitting up. To gauge how much your baby may be spitting up, you can pour a teaspoon of milk onto the counter and compare it to the amount your baby spits up. The amounts are probably similar. Spit-up doesn't typically upset babies. In fact, they may not even notice it. If your baby seems agitated or in pain during or after spitting up, or if you think the volume is more than an ounce, consult your pediatrician.

Hiccups

As your milk volume increases and your baby transfers a larger quantity of milk, she may start to hiccup after feedings. This is normal and usually means she had a good feeding and her tummy is full. Hiccups often bother baby's caregiver more than they bother baby.

Growth Spurts

During growths spurts, which usually last about two to four days, your baby will want to eat more frequently due to rapid physical growth. Your milk supply will increase during this time because of baby's increasing demand. Continue to feed your baby as often as she wants. You may notice that your baby sleeps longer for a few days at the end of a growth spurt. The chart to the right shows the typical ages for growth spurts. Remember that your baby's growth spurts may not exactly follow this pattern, so if she suddenly wants to eat more frequently at a different age, follow her lead. Some moms worry that the increased demand means they do not have enough milk for their babies. This is rarely the case. In fact, supplementing with formula during a growth spurt can interrupt the feedback between baby and breast that will ensure your milk supply increases to match her demand.

Ages for Typical Growth Spurts
9-10 days
3-4 weeks
6 weeks
3 months
6 months
9 months

Gas

Many newborns are gassy, due in part to their frequent feedings. Most babies pass gas regularly without any discomfort. If your baby shows signs of discomfort after feedings by arching her back or lifting her legs, she is probably having trouble passing gas.

To address uncomfortable gassiness:

- Take frequent breaks while breastfeeding to burp baby.
- Lean back after baby latches to help slow the milk flow.
- Track foods you eat that may be upsetting baby's tummy by keeping a food diary.
- Lie baby on her back and move her legs like bicycle pedals.
- Lie baby on her tummy (good opportunity for tummy time).
- Do gentle circular tummy massage, going clockwise around baby's navel.
- Hold baby with gentle pressure on her tummy.
- Hold baby upright while you bounce on exercise ball.

If these methods do not help your baby feel more comfortable, ask your pediatrician about other remedies, such as over-the-counter or prescription medicines.

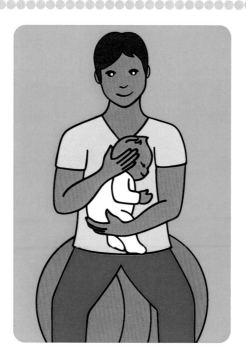

Uneven Milk Supply

It is not uncommon for moms to produce more milk from one breast than the other. For many moms, the right breast produces more. This may be due to differing amounts of mammary tissue in each breast. It can also be due to mom's or baby's breast preference, leading to frequent feeding on that side and thus increasing its milk volume. Breast preference might result from your baby preferring to be on one side versus the other, which may match how she was positioned in utero. You can attempt to even out your milk supply by starting every feeding on the side that produces less for a few weeks or until your milk supply becomes more even, as baby typically feeds more vigorously on the first side when she is hungrier. Some moms pump the lesser producing side after feedings temporarily, for about five minutes, to encourage more milk production. If you are struggling with low milk supply, see page 74 for more information.

Oversupply/Overactive Letdown

It may seem that having too much milk is a great problem, but it can be difficult to manage. Babies of moms with an oversupply may have greenish poops, may be gassy and fussy, and may want to nurse more frequently because they are receiving less of the fatty milk from the end of a feeding.

Some ways to address oversupply include:

- Feed baby on only one side per feeding.
- Use the laid-back breastfeeding position so baby works against gravity to remove milk.
- Insert green cabbage leaves in bra for short periods of time (no more than 20 minutes, a few times a day).
- Take herbs that are known to reduce supply (e.g., sage and peppermint).

Another, sometimes related, problem is a forceful or overactive letdown. If your baby latches off the breast, coughing, choking or gagging, you may have an overactive letdown. You will likely notice milk spraying from your breast when baby latches off suddenly.

To help with a forceful/overactive letdown:

- Manually express milk during the initial letdown and wait to latch baby when the flow slows.
- Burb baby frequently during and after feedings.
- Keep baby's mouth and nipple/areola dry when attempting to latch or relatch.

If you have an oversupply of milk and you have pumped milk that you can't use, consider donating it to a milk bank (www.hmbana.org) or to one of several milk sharing networks like Eats on Feets (www.eatsonfeets.org) or Human Milk 4 Human Babies (www.hm4hb.net).

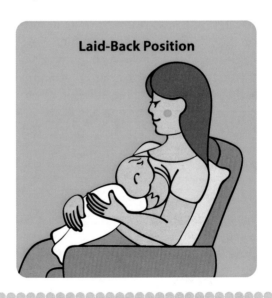

Laid-Back Position

Evening Fussiness

Babies are notoriously fussy in the evening, right around dinnertime, when the house is bustling with noise and food preparation. During what many parents call the "witching hour," babies often want to feed more frequently. This may be because mom's milk supply is lower at this time of day and/or because baby may be overtired and overstimulated. Breastfeeding during fussy periods calms baby and can also be calming for mom if she is able to relax and breastfeed.

Other reasons for baby's fussiness and desire for frequent or cluster feeding at any time of day are:

- Illness
- Teething
- Growth spurts
- Overstimulation

In general, it's best to feed your baby on demand through these fussy times. However, if you suspect that your baby is fussy from gas, it's best not to feed so frequently. Some babies merely want to comfort suck and will latch off and get upset when the milk starts flowing because they aren't actually hungry. If you think this may be the case and your baby is gaining weight appropriately, you can offer a pacifier so your baby can suck for comfort. Your baby will let you know if she's genuinely hungry by spitting out the pacifier and crying.

Crying in the Closet

My daughter had what some call "evening colic" during the first three months. She would cry inconsolably from about 5 p.m. to 8 p.m. most nights. When my husband returned home from work, he would wear her in a front carrier and go into our dark walk-in closet, as he bounced her and made shushing noises. The dark, quiet room helped to calm her down and she would often fall asleep on him. We figured out she was probably just overstimulated from the day's activities.

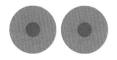

CHAPTER 7
UNCOMMON PROBLEMS

Although the following problems are rare, you may encounter one or more during your breastfeeding experience. These should be addressed as soon as possible by a lactation consultant, pediatrician, and/or obstetrician. You may find it challenging to work through them, but none of these problems should end your breastfeeding relationship with your baby if you have a good support system in place.

Thrush

Thrush is an overgrowth of yeast on the nipple and areola. Typically, thrush is characterized by a burning, stinging, or stabbing pain on mom's nipples during and between feedings. The nipples and areola may appear irritated and small white patches may be present. Baby may or may not have symptoms, which can include white patches on baby's tongue and inner cheeks that do not wipe away with a cloth. Some babies also develop a dotted diaper rash that does not go away with normal diaper creams. In this case, you may need to use a topical antifungal cream on the rash, although you should check with your pediatrician before using any medication. It is not uncommon for moms to develop thrush after taking antibiotics, either before, during, or after the birth, because antibiotics kill the beneficial bacteria that help to prevent an overgrowth of yeast. Contact your pediatrician and obstetrician if you suspect that you or your baby has developed thrush. The usual treatment is an oral antifungal for mom and topical treatment for inside baby's mouth. Mom and baby should be treated at the same time to completely address the problem. Ideally, treatment should continue for one week after symptoms disappear. During thrush treatment, be sure to clean and sterilize anything that comes into contact with baby's mouth or your breastmilk daily. This includes bottles, pacifiers, and pump parts. If you have fresh milk that was pumped while you and your baby are being treated for thrush, it is safe to offer it to baby. If you have frozen milk that was pumped during a thrush outbreak, scald the milk first and let it cool before offering it to baby.

Plugged Ducts

A plugged duct occurs when a small amount of breastmilk hardens inside a milk duct, causing pain and restricting milk flow. A plugged duct feels like a firm, pea-sized lump under the skin that does not become smaller after a feeding. Plugged ducts often occur when intervals between feedings lengthen, such as when baby starts sleeping longer at night. They can also be caused by wearing bras that are too tight or have an underwire. Try to move the hardened milk through the duct as soon as possible. If not cleared, the duct can become infected, possibly leading to mastitis. Applying a warm compress on the site of the plug can help loosen it before feeding or pumping on the affected side. Once the feeding starts, rub your finger firmly over the plugged duct in a circular motion, trying to move the plug toward the nipple. If that doesn't work, try taking a warm bath, submerging your entire breast and nipple for at least ten minutes while doing circular massage. Feeding directly after a bath or shower can help. You can also try using the vibrating end of an electric toothbrush or a mini-massager to break up the plug. If you are still having trouble moving the plugged milk through, you may be able to find a healthcare professional (e.g., physical therapist or chiropractor) in your area who uses ultrasound therapy to clear the plugged duct. Moms who experience frequent and recurrent plugged ducts may benefit from taking a supplement called lecithin to help prevent future plugged ducts. Typical dosage is 1200 mg. three or four times per day. Plugged ducts can temporarily reduce milk supply on the affected breast.

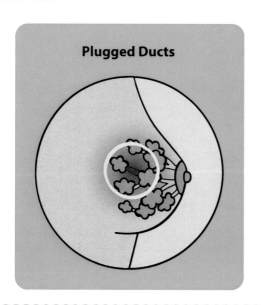

Plugged Ducts

There are white things floating in my bath water!

I remember working with a mom who was struggling with a plugged duct. I suggested she take a warm bath, submerging her breasts and nipples in water for ten minutes and then doing circular massage over the plug, trying to move it toward the nipple. After her bath, she asked me what the little white things floating in her bath water were. I explained that they were pieces of hardened milk that had been clogging her milk duct.

Mastitis

Mastitis is an infection of the breast tissue occurring in one or both breasts. Although typically caused by a plugged duct that has not cleared, it can also be caused by bacteria from baby's mouth entering mom's breast through a cracked nipple. Mastitis may occur at any point during breastfeeding. Early symptoms include a general feeling of achiness, flu-like symptoms, breast pain and redness, and a warm feeling on the exterior of the infected breast. Some moms also develop a fever of 101 degrees Fahrenheit or higher. There is no reason to stop breastfeeding if you develop mastitis. Milk supply on the affected breast may decrease during the infection.

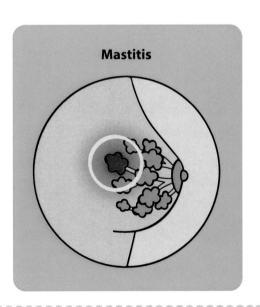

Mastitis

You may be able to prevent a full-blown case of mastitis by trying some of these techniques within the first 24 hours of symptoms developing:

- Rest for mom (treat yourself as if you have the flu)
- Frequent feedings, especially on the infected breast
- Warm compresses on breast before feedings
- Cold compresses on breast after feedings
- Vitamin C, Echinacea, Zinc supplements for mom
- Over-the-counter fever-reducing medicine

Mastitis that does not resolve within 24 hours should be treated with oral antibiotics prescribed by your obstetrician or primary care doctor. It is perfectly safe to continue breastfeeding while taking antibiotics, and your baby will not need any treatment. Taking probiotics during your antibiotic treatment to replace the beneficial bacteria in your body may be helpful.

Milk Blebs/Milk Blisters

A milk bleb or blister is a clogged milk pore on your nipple. Each nipple has approximately ten pores for breastmilk to pass through. Occasionally, skin will grow over a nipple pore, causing milk to become trapped underneath. This may look like a white dot under the skin and can feel quite painful. To alleviate the pain and help the nipple pore to open, you can use a warm compress directly on the nipple for about ten minutes prior to breastfeeding. You also can try soaking your nipple in a bowl of very warm water mixed with a tablespoon of Epsom salt before breastfeeding. Between feedings, put some olive oil on a cotton ball and place it directly on your nipple, covering it with a breast pad inside your bra. All of these treatments will help to soften the skin. Once the skin has been softened, gently rub the nipple area with a wet washcloth to try to open the pore. When it eventually opens, don't be surprised if the milk appears somewhat hardened. It is perfectly safe for your baby to ingest this hardened milk if the blister opens during a feeding. If you have tried these treatments and the blister still won't open, contact your obstetrician or primary care doctor to have it released. Introducing a needle into your nipple can cause infection and is best done by a licensed medical professional. (See next page for illustration.)

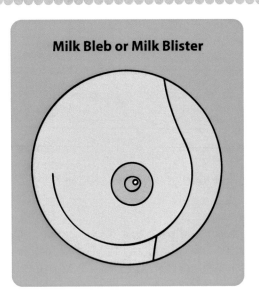

Milk Bleb or Milk Blister

Tongue and Lip Tie

Tongue tie and lip tie are anatomical conditions that may affect breastfeeding. A baby is considered tongue-tied when the skin that connects the tongue to the base of the mouth (frenulum) is tight, restricting normal movement of the tongue. A lip tie is when the skin that connects baby's upper lip to his gums is tight and low on the gum line, sometimes as far down as the bottom of the gum line where his teeth will eventually grow in. These ties can restrict the movement that is necessary to breastfeed effectively, inhibiting baby from transferring an adequate amount of milk and causing severe nipple pain for mom.

Symptoms of tongue and/or lip tie:

• Visible string-like skin under baby's tongue or top lip
• Severely sore, cracked, and/or bleeding nipples
• Long, slow, sleepy, and painful feedings
• Slow weight gain despite frequent feedings
• Excessive spit up and gas
• Decreasing milk supply

If you suspect that your baby has a tongue or lip tie and you are experiencing any of the symptoms above, contact a lactation consultant, pediatrician, pediatric dentist, or pediatric ear, nose, and throat doctor. For more information on tongue and lip ties, visit the Tongue Tie website (tonguetie.net/breastfeeding/).

Nursing Strike

Sometimes a previously happily breastfed baby will suddenly refuse to breastfeed. This is called a nursing strike and it can be upsetting to mom as she worries about her baby's nutritional needs as well as the lack of breast stimulation, which can diminish her milk supply. It's never a good idea to attempt to force your baby to breastfeed during a nursing strike. We can only *encourage* baby to return to the breast. Most babies younger than a year old will resume breastfeeding within a week. If your baby is older than a year and the strike lasts longer than a week, she may be showing signs of readiness to wean. (See page 100 for more on weaning.) During a nursing strike, pump both breasts for fifteen minutes at the times your baby normally breastfeeds to maintain your milk supply. Feed him with a bottle or cup until he resumes breastfeeding.

Common causes of nursing strikes:

- Teething (may be painful to breastfeed)
- Illness (causing lack of appetite)
- Ear infection (may be painful to breastfeed)
- Cold or stuffy nose (baby can't breathe through nose while feeding)
- Upsetting incident at breast, like mom reacting strongly after baby bit her
- Plugged duct or mastitis, limiting mom's milk flow
- Pregnancy (milk may taste different or decrease in volume)

Ways to encourage baby to breastfeed:

- Offer breast when baby is sleepy (before or just after sleep).
- Offer breast when baby is distracted.
- Attend breastfeeding support group where baby will see other babies nursing.
- Provide lots of skin to skin contact.
- Get in bed with baby, without a shirt on, and cuddle.
- Take bath with baby.

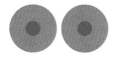

Bottle Refusal

Ideally your baby will have been drinking milk from a bottle at least three times a week, starting at around four to six weeks of age, so he gets accustomed to bottle feeding. If baby has not been getting regular bottles and is an enthusiastic breast feeder, he may not want to take a bottle when you need him to, for example, when you return to work.

Some ways to coax a reluctant baby to take a bottle:

- Have someone other than mom offer the bottle. Ideally mom will not be in the same room.
- Hold baby in a position different than when baby is breastfed.
- Make sure the milk is warm enough. Baby is used to breastmilk that is approximately 98.6 degrees Fahrenheit.
- Offer the bottle when baby is a bit sleepy.
- Offer a bottle about thirty minutes after a regular feeding time. Often babies will take this dessert feeding more readily than when the bottle substitutes for a full meal.
- Have partner or other caregiver hold baby on their lap, facing out with some kind of toy distracting him. Offer bottle once baby seems interested in the distraction.

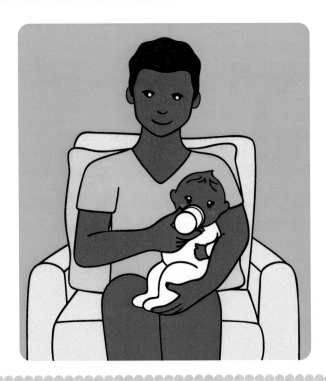

Most babies will eventually take breastmilk from a bottle if mom is not around. If baby continues to refuse the bottle, you can try cup feeding. Hold the baby upright in your lap. Offer milk in a small cup, letting baby lap up the milk slowly. Take breaks to allow him to swallow. Some babies go straight to a cup after breastfeeding and skip right over the bottle phase.

Biting

Biting is a natural concern for breastfeeding moms. However, babies do not actually use their teeth when breastfeeding. When a baby is actively sucking, his tongue covers his bottom gums and teeth. When your baby is teething, he may clamp down during or near the end of a feeding in an effort to soothe his sore gums. One way to prevent biting is to pay close attention to when baby's sucking slows down toward the end of a feeding. Notice as soon as he stops sucking and remove him from the breast before he has the chance to teethe on your nipple. If your baby bites while breastfeeding, take him off the breast and tell him "No" in a calm but firm voice. Wait a few minutes before resuming breastfeeding. Repeat this process if the biting continues so baby gets the message that biting is not okay. You can minimize baby's inclination to bite or clamp down if he is teething by offering a cold washcloth or teething ring for baby to suck on before feeding him.

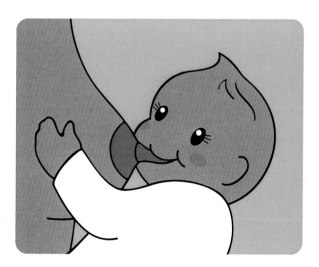

CHAPTER 8
MOM'S DIET AND MILK SUPPLY

The most important thing you can do to maintain a healthy milk supply is to feed your baby frequently. This translates to feeding on demand (whenever your baby shows interest in eating) and at least every three to four hours, depending on your baby's age. The more demand there is for milk through breast stimulation, the more your body will respond by continuing to make milk.

Mom's Diet

Just as you did during pregnancy, you will want to eat a nutritious, balanced diet while breastfeeding, including protein, carbs, healthy fats, and a variety of fruits and vegetables. The good news is that you no longer need to avoid foods like soft cheeses, sushi, certain fish, and processed meats, as you did during your pregnancy. You'll probably feel quite hungry; you will burn approximately 500 calories per day just from breastfeeding! This isn't a time to diet. Your body will naturally shed those extra pregnancy pounds. Doctors recommend that you continue taking a prenatal vitamin or multivitamin to supplement your diet during your entire breastfeeding experience.

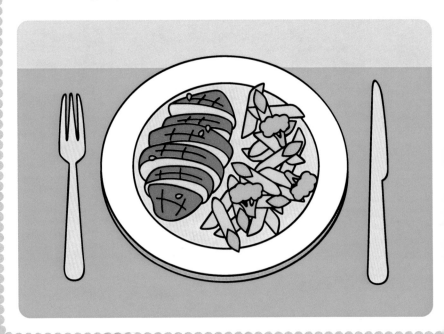

Should You Avoid Any Foods?

Some breastfeeding moms worry about how the foods they eat will affect their babies. However, you don't need to avoid any particular foods when breastfeeding. Babies all over the world breastfeed while their moms eat everything from curry and chili to broccoli and beans. In fact, the wider the variety of foods that you eat while breastfeeding, the less picky your child will be when she starts eating solids, since she will have been exposed to so many different flavors through your breastmilk. Having said that, it *is* possible for your baby to be sensitive to certain foods you eat. It typically takes at least four hours for the food you consume to make it into your milk. If your baby becomes unusually fussy or gassy, think about what you ate earlier that day. If you suspect your baby might be sensitive to a particular food, you can test your theory by eating that food again. If eating the same food leads to the same symptoms, try avoiding that food for a few weeks. You can then try reintroducing that food into your diet as your baby gets a little older. She may be able to tolerate it as her digestive system matures. Remember that babies are naturally gassy. As tempting as it is to find a straightforward explanation, mom's diet rarely causes gassiness. If your baby is extremely gassy and fussy all the time, you might want to start eliminating foods that can cause issues for some babies, one at a time, to see if that helps. One food group that lactation consultants suggest eliminating first is dairy, including milk, cheese, yogurt, ice cream, and other milk-based products. Note that it may take up to three weeks for dairy to completely leave your system.

Snacks

You will feel surprisingly hungry while breastfeeding and your meal prep time will be limited, as you'll be busy feeding and caring for your new baby. Keep a supply of quick, healthy snacks next to the place that you nurse most frequently. That way you can grab a quick snack while feeding, to keep your energy up and your body nourished.

Some ideas for quick, healthy snacks are:

- Nutrition bars
- Nuts/trail mix
- Granola

- Fruits and vegetables
- Cheese and crackers
- Yogurt

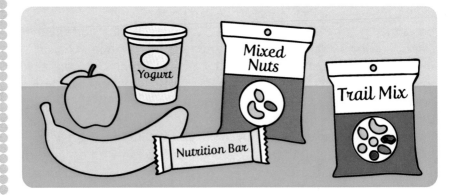

Water Intake

Staying adequately hydrated while breastfeeding helps to maintain a healthy milk supply. You probably will feel quite thirsty, so keep a water bottle handy and drink to thirst.

Caffeine

Although avoiding caffeine was recommended during your pregnancy, you can now enjoy that cup of coffee or tea you've been longing for. It is perfectly safe to drink one or two cups of a caffeinated beverage each day. Caffeine does not typically have any noticeable effect on babies. However, if you notice that your baby is irritable or is having difficulty sleeping, reduce your caffeine intake or stop drinking it altogether, and try again when your baby is a little older.

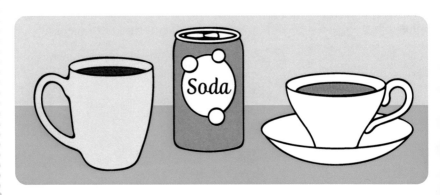

Alcohol

Most doctors agree that it's fine to have an occasional glass of wine or a beer when you are breastfeeding. The important factor to consider is timing. The level of alcohol in breastmilk is the same as the level of alcohol in your bloodstream. It takes about two hours for one serving of alcohol to leave your bloodstream AND your breastmilk. Because babies breastfeed about every three hours, you can time alcohol consumption for immediately after a feeding so that the alcohol will naturally be out of your system before the next feeding. Be sure to consider the size of the drink. The two-hour time frame is based on a 12-ounce bottle of beer, a 5-ounce glass of wine, or a mixed drink that contains about 1.5 ounces of alcohol. You can find calculators online to help you determine specifics for you, based on your body weight. If your baby awakens earlier than expected and you are concerned that alcohol is still present in your breastmilk, feed her previously pumped milk. Then pump both breasts for fifteen minutes and discard the milk. Wait to breastfeed regularly at the next feeding. Another option is to manually express a small amount of breastmilk and use test strips that screen for alcohol in your milk so you know whether or not it is safe to breastfeed. (UpSpring Baby: www.upspringbaby.com) You may have heard that drinking beer can increase your milk supply. The ingredients in beer that may be responsible for the increase are barley, hops, and brewer's yeast-not the alcohol. These ingredients are also in non-alcoholic beer, which is a much safer option while breastfeeding. If you are going to an event where you know you will be drinking for an extended period of time (for example, a wedding or a party), you'll need to pump both breasts for fifteen minutes about every three hours to avoid leaking, engorgement, and plugged ducts. Because the milk you pump during this time will contain alcohol, you should discard it. This is sometimes referred to as "pumping and dumping." The only thing that will remove alcohol from your breastmilk is time.

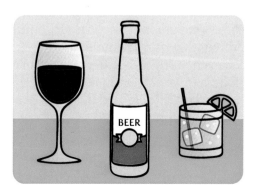

Medication

At some point during your breastfeeding journey, you may need to take medication. Most are completely safe, but check with your doctor before taking any medication. If you have a cold or sinus infection, it's best to avoid any medications that will dry up mucous membranes, as they may significantly decrease your milk supply. For thorough information on medication safety while breastfeeding, visit Mommy Meds (www.mommymeds.com).

Low Milk Supply

Despite eating a well-balanced diet and drinking lots of water, some moms are simply not able to make enough breastmilk for their babies. This can happen for a variety of reasons, such as infrequent feedings, poor latch, hormonal imbalances, or not having enough glandular tissue to make and store breastmilk. Many moms have been successful in increasing their milk supply by increasing the number of feedings per day, pumping after feedings for extra stimulation, taking herbs and, in rare cases, taking medication. A lactation consultant can help you come up with a plan to increase your milk supply. The most important thing to ensure is that your baby gets fed, regardless of how.

Galactagogues

Galactagogues are foods or herbs that have been shown to increase milk supply for many breastfeeding moms. Some foods that may help boost a marginal milk supply are oatmeal, almonds, carrots, sweet potatoes, apricots, and salmon. Because they're part of a healthy diet anyway, it can't hurt to try them. If you are struggling to make enough milk for your baby, you may also consider trying one or more herbal supplements. I recommend trying one at a time, as you may find one particular herb that works best for you. You can eat these in their natural form or take them in a concentrated capsule or tincture. Some products contain a combination of herbs that may be beneficial. You can even purchase cookies that contain galactagogues that claim to increase milk supply. If they don't work, at least you can enjoy a much-deserved treat. Check with your doctor before taking any herbal supplements.

Some of the most common herbal galactagogues are:

- Brewer's yeast
- Goat's rue
- Moringa

- Blessed Thistle
- Fennel
- Nettle

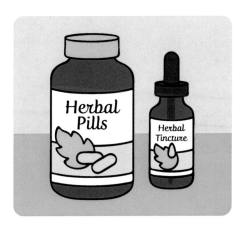

Supplementation

Babies who not gaining enough weight will need to receive extra milk (supplement) in addition to the milk they get from the breast, in order to meet their nutritional needs. The ideal supplement is breastmilk that is pumped in between breastfeeding sessions. If mom does not have any extra breastmilk, donor milk or formula can be used. You can offer the supplement in several ways, depending on the age of the baby and how frequently you need to supplement.

Ways to offer supplement:

- At the breast with a feeding tube, while breastfeeding
- Soft syringe
- Small cup
- Bottle

If possible, it's best to delay the use of a bottle in the early weeks postpartum because some babies develop a preference for its faster flow. If you choose to use a bottle for supplementation, see page 84 to learn how to pace the feeding so that the bottle flows similarly to the breast. The most important thing is that your baby gets enough breastmilk or formula to meet her nutritional needs. Contact your pediatrician or lactation consultant for guidance on an appropriate feeding method and amount.

CHAPTER 9
PUMPING AND BOTTLE FEEDING

If breastfeeding is going well in the first few weeks, there is no reason to begin pumping your breasts for extra milk. However, if your baby isn't latching or you are offering supplemental feedings in addition to or in place of breastfeeding, then you will need to begin pumping to collect milk and to protect your milk supply. There are many different breast pumps on the market, varying greatly in style, price, and effectiveness. Most moms receive a breast pump through their insurance company. Investigate your insurance plan's pump options during your pregnancy so you will have the pump ready to use, should you need it. You can also purchase a manual pump or rent a hospital-grade pump, depending on your individual needs.

Types of Pumps	Best Used For
Manual Pump	Relieving engorgement or for occasional bottle
Personal Electric Pump	Occasional bottle or pumping when away from baby
Hospital-Grade Pump	Protecting milk supply when baby gets supplement

Manual pumps are the least expensive and are best used for relieving engorgement either during the first few weeks or anytime your breasts feel uncomfortably full. These pumps have no motor. Instead, mom generates suction using her hand to pump milk from one breast at a time. Electric pumps rely on a motor to create suction and are perfect for pumping milk for future bottle feedings or when mom has to be away from baby. Many moms carry these pumps to work each day.

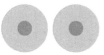

Although there are electric pumps intended for single-breast pumping, it's best to use a double electric pump to pump both breasts simultaneously, yielding more milk. A hospital-grade pump has an efficient motor that effectively removes milk and protects mom's milk supply when baby is not able to latch or is receiving an extra supplement, especially during the first month. You can rent one from a hospital, birth center, or breastfeeding supply store. Most insurance companies will cover the cost of a hospital-grade pump rental, especially if your baby isn't latching, so be sure to get a receipt to submit with your insurance claim.

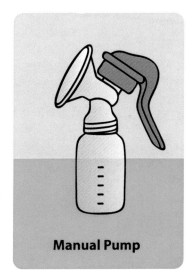

Manual Pump

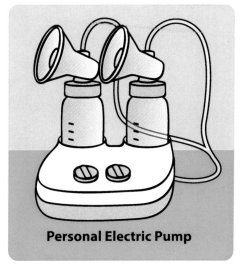

Personal Electric Pump

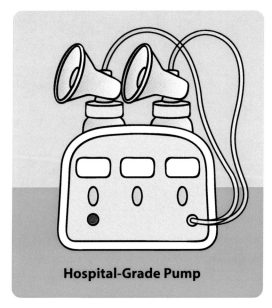

Hospital-Grade Pump

Pump Kits

Most electric pumps come with all of the parts you'll need. These include the tubing, flanges, valves, and bottles. Before using your pump for the first time, follow the manufacturer's instructions, which usually recommend sterilizing all of the pump parts that come into contact with your breastmilk. There is no need to sterilize the tubing, as only air moves through it while pumping. If the tubing gets wet inside, replace it to avoid mold growth.

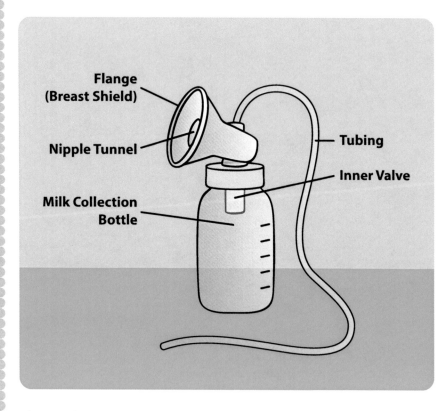

Flange (Breast Shield)

Nipple Tunnel

Milk Collection Bottle

Tubing

Inner Valve

Flange Size

Make sure you use the appropriate flange (breast shield) size when pumping. Flange sizes range from 17 mm to 36 mm. Most pumps come with 24 mm size flanges, which fit the majority of women. If necessary, you can purchase larger or smaller flanges for your pump depending on the size of your nipples. While you are pumping, your nipple should move freely inside the cone part of the flange without touching the plastic sides. Your nipples may increase in size while you pump, so make sure that they move freely throughout the pumping session.

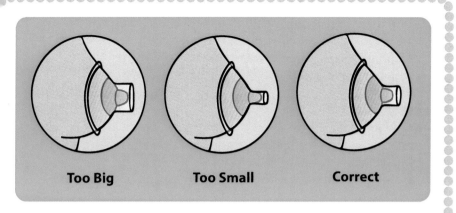

| Too Big | Too Small | Correct |

When to Pump

The decision about when to start pumping will depend on your particular situation. If your baby is exclusively breastfeeding and gaining weight, it's preferable to wait to start pumping until your baby is between four and six weeks old when you will introduce a bottle. By this time, breastfeeding should be well established and your baby will still be open to a new feeding method. If you are offering any additional milk to your baby, either in place of or in addition to breastfeeding, you'll need to pump both breasts for fifteen minutes, whenever your baby receives a supplement. This works to replace the additional demand, in order to protect your milk supply. Ask your pediatrician or a lactation consultant about specific supplement amounts and pumping duration. If you are pumping while away from your baby, the general rule is to pump both breasts at the same time about every three hours for fifteen minutes. This helps to protect your milk supply and prevent engorgement and plugged ducts. You do not have to time your pumping sessions with your baby's exact feeding times. Approximately every three hours is sufficient. Depending on your situation, you may find yourself pumping in an empty office space, a mothers' room at a store, or even in your car, while parked or even while driving!

How to Pump

When you are ready to pump, sit in a comfortable space and attach all the parts from your pump kit to your pump. Every pump is a little different, but most have an on/off switch, a suction setting, and a speed setting.

- Turn the pump on and make sure the suction and speed settings are set to a comfortable level. Some pumps adjust the speed automatically, so refer to the manufacturer's instruction guide for your particular pump.
- Position the flanges on your breasts, carefully centering the cones over your nipples.
- Hold the bottles with your hands and gently push in toward your breasts. Make sure that the flanges fit snugly and that no air exits the flanges.
- Slowly increase the suction but go only as high as you can while remaining comfortable. The sensation should feel like a gentle tugging and should not be painful. Any pain you feel will inhibit your milk flow.
- If your pump does not adjust the speed automatically, increase the speed as much as you can, making sure you don't experience any pain. This fast setting mimics your baby sucking quickly at the beginning of a breastfeeding session, as he signals the milk to let down or begin to flow.
- Once milk starts flowing from both nipples, decrease the speed by about one-third and maintain this speed setting while milk is flowing.
- When your milk flow slows down or stops, increase the speed again to see if you can stimulate another letdown.
- Continue pumping for the amount of time suggested by your lactation consultant or pediatrician. The duration will vary depending on your pumping goals, whether your baby is latching, and how much supplement you are offering.

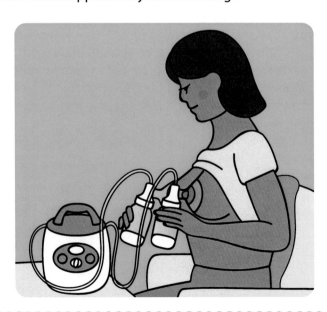

Hands-On Pumping

Although breast pumps do a great job removing milk, moms typically extract less milk using a pump than their baby does when breastfeeding. This is because moms have a greater hormonal response to their babies than to a machine. Hands-free pumping bras hold the flanges and bottles in place, leaving your hands free to massage your breasts while pumping, which can help increase the amount of milk removed. Use your hands to massage different parts of the breast, moving your hands in a small circular motion over any lumpy or dense areas. You will learn the spots to massage that help to yield the most milk. If you still feel dense or lumpy spots beneath the skin after pumping, you can manually express without the pump to extract even more milk. (See page 15 on Manual Expression.)

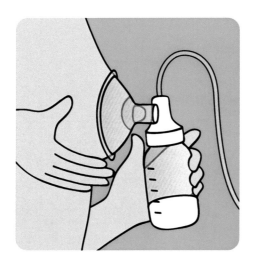

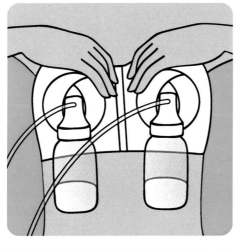

Pumping for Extra Milk

With all the breastfeeding you are doing, you may wonder when you should pump to collect extra milk for bottle feeding without depleting your baby's next meal. Levels of prolactin (the hormone that produces milk) are highest from the middle of the night through the morning hours, making this the most effective time to pump in between feedings. You should be able to pump a sufficient amount of milk without significantly reducing the milk your baby will receive at his next meal. To do this, wait thirty minutes after a first morning feeding to give your breasts time to replenish their supply. Then pump both breasts at the same time for fifteen minutes. Breastfeed normally at the next feeding. Another option is to pump several times throughout the day after a feeding, particularly if your baby has a smaller meal or drains only one breast. You can chill and combine small amounts of pumped milk to make up a full feeding.

Cleaning Pump Parts

It's important to keep all of your pump parts clean in between pumping sessions. Follow the manufacturer's guidelines, which usually suggest washing all parts (except tubing) with warm soapy water and letting them air dry. This goes for bottles as well. Make sure to separate all of the parts when washing (including the valve) in order to avoid mold growth.

Breastmilk Storage Guidelines

Breastmilk can be stored in milk storage bags, bottles, or any container that has been cleaned ahead of time. If you plan to freeze breastmilk, pour it into a bag or bottle and leave a little room for the milk to expand during the freezing process. Write the date on the container, since you should always use the oldest milk first. You may want to store some of your breastmilk in smaller amounts for times when your baby needs a snack and not a full feeding while you are away. You can store breastmilk in the refrigerator for up to six days and in the freezer for up to six months. Do not combine milk from different pumping sessions until both portions are the same temperature. If freezing, place the container of milk in the larger part of the freezer toward the back and not in the freezer door. If you know that you will not be using the milk that you pumped within six days, place it directly into the freezer. Freezing breastmilk does destroy some of its immune properties, but it is still completely safe and healthy to feed to your baby.

Breastmilk Storage Guidelines		
Storage Type	Freshly Expressed Breastmilk	Thawed Breastmilk
Room Temp	Up to 6 Hours	Do Not Store
Cooler Bag with Ice	24 Hours	Do Not Store
Fridge	Up to 6 Days	24 Hours
Fridge Freezer	Up to 6 Months	Never Refreeze Thawed Breastmilk
Deep Freezer	Up to 8 Months	Never Refreeze Thawed Breastmilk

Preparing Breastmilk

To defrost frozen breastmilk, place the container of milk in the refrigerator overnight. If you need to defrost the milk quickly, place the container of milk in a larger container of warm water, or run warm water over the container in the sink. You can warm refrigerated breastmilk the same way, or you can use a bottle warmer. Some babies prefer their bottled milk to be warm while others will drink pumped milk regardless of its temperature. Once the milk is thawed, you may notice a separation as the higher fat milk rises to the top. Gently swirl (don't shake) the bottle to combine the separated milk before offering to your baby. Never microwave breastmilk, as it destroys essential nutrients and heats unevenly, making it unsafe for your baby to drink. Aim to use thawed milk within 24 hours of defrosting. If your baby doesn't finish a previously thawed bottle of breastmilk, you can store it in the fridge and reheat it again for the next feeding within three hours. Never refreeze thawed breastmilk. Note that guidelines for storing formula are different, especially regarding partially finished bottles, which should be discarded. For more information on storing and preparing breastmilk, visit The Centers for Disease Control website (www.cdc.breastfeeding/recommendations/handling_breastmilk.htm).

Bottles

There are many different types of bottles on the market, varying in shape, size, style, and material. You'll want to look for one that best mimics your baby's mouth shape and tongue movement while breastfeeding. Compare the different sizes of base widths and nipple teat lengths, and choose one that is medium sized in both cases. This type of bottle will encourage your baby to open his mouth wide and grasp a good portion of the nipple teat and base, which is most similar to breastfeeding. You may want to purchase a few different bottle styles to see which one you and your baby like best. An important factor when choosing a bottle nipple is making sure the flow is as slow as possible (size 0 or 1). You will usually find slow-flow nipples on smaller bottles, labeled for newborns. For breastfed babies, you don't typically need to increase the nipple flow size as your baby grows, since it's best to maintain a slow flow that is similar to breastfeeding, regardless of baby's age.

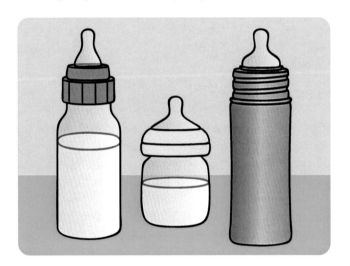

Bottle Feeding

A good time to introduce a bottle is when your baby reaches about four to six weeks of age. By this time, breastfeeding is typically well established and your baby should still be open to an alternative feeding method. Offer a bottle at least three times a week to make sure baby remains interested and will accept a bottle when mom isn't around. To make sure your baby will happily take milk from both your breast and a bottle, you will want to pace the bottle feeding to replicate the flow of milk when breastfeeding. This method, often referred to as "paced bottle feeding," is a relaxed and respectful way to bottle feed your baby that allows him to drink at his own pace. He can take sucking breaks without having the milk pour quickly into his mouth. Otherwise, he is forced to continue sucking and swallowing quickly and repetitively, causing stress and leading to increased gas and discomfort after feedings. Despite how stressful quick bottle feeding can be for babies, some learn to expect this faster flow and get fussy when breastfeeding, due to the slower flow of milk. Therefore, it is important to bottle feed slowly to protect the breastfeeding relationship.

How to pace a bottle feeding:

- Hold baby upright while holding the bottle horizontal.
- Stroke baby's top lip and wait for him to open his mouth wide, just like he does when latching onto the breast.
- Insert the bottle nipple all the way into his mouth so his lips rest on the nipple base.
- Continue holding the bottle horizontally, allowing the nipple to fill halfway with milk.
- Let baby drink at his own pace and let him pause anytime he wants.
- Burp the baby halfway through and at the end of the feeding.

Using paced bottle feeding, it should take baby about five minutes to drink an ounce of milk. Therefore, a three-ounce bottle feeding should take about fifteen minutes. If you notice your baby is drinking from a bottle much faster, revisit the suggestions above. If your baby does not finish a bottle of breastmilk, you can place it in the refrigerator and use it for the next feeding within three hours.

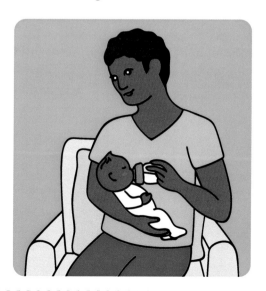

How Much Milk to Offer

Babies will often take the full amount of milk offered in a bottle, regardless of how hungry they are. This is because of their high suck need in the first few months. Offer an appropriate amount of milk to avoid tummy discomfort and overfeeding. If you are offering milk in a bottle, you can use the following equation to determine approximately how much milk to offer. Note that these amounts are too much to offer a baby less than ten days old.

Daily Milk Requirements by Weight

Baby's current weight multiplied by 2.5 = total ounces per day

$$\frac{\text{Total ounces per day}}{\text{\# of feedings in a 24 hour period}} = \text{Approximate ounces per feeding}$$

Example:
8 lbs. x 2.5 = 20 oz. per day

$$\frac{20 \text{ oz.}}{10 \text{ feedings per day}} = 2 \text{ oz. per bottle feeding}$$

Therefore, an eight-pound baby who eats ten times per day needs about two ounces of milk for a replacement bottle. The amount of breastmilk transferred in any particular breastfeeding session will vary, so use this as a guideline for bottle feeding. Once baby is two or three months old, the amount of milk he takes per feeding will remain about the same throughout the rest of his breastfeeding experience. This is because milk composition changes over time to meet baby's developmental needs and because nutrition levels are not related to milk volume.

Bottle Refusal

Sometimes breastfeeding is going so well that babies reject taking milk in a bottle. To avoid this, offer baby at least three bottles each week once breastfeeding is established to keep him interested in bottle feeding. It's never a good idea to try to force your baby to take a bottle.

Suggestions to encourage baby to take a bottle:

- Have someone other than mom offer the bottle.
- Don't have mom in the same room when bottle is offered.
- Sit in a different spot than where baby typically breastfeeds.
- Hold baby in a position that's different from a breastfeeding position.
- Make sure milk in the bottle is warm enough (approximately 98 degrees Fahrenheit).
- Offer a small amount of milk in a bottle about thirty minutes after breastfeeding as a little dessert, without the pressure of getting him to take a whole feeding.
- Take baby out of the home, where he is likely to see other babies drinking from a bottle.

My baby won't take a bottle!

One of the moms I worked with had a three-month-old baby and was planning to return to work soon. Although her baby had taken a bottle a few times when it was offered at six weeks of age, she had stopped offering a bottle regularly since the breastfeeding was going so well. Now she was frantic because her baby would no longer take a bottle, and she was worried that her baby wouldn't take it while she was at work. We worked together to get her baby to successfully take a bottle from dad while mom was out of the room. We were all relieved when her baby ended up taking bottles regularly, without a problem, once she returned to work.

CHAPTER 10
RETURNING TO WORK

Returning to work after having a baby can bring mixed emotions. Some moms feel terribly guilty about leaving their baby in someone else's care, while others look forward to rejoining the world of adults and their chosen profession. Pumping at work can be time-consuming and stressful, as you try to balance your work responsibilities with a regular pumping schedule. If you feel overwhelmed, try to remember that this extra demand on your time is temporary. You will be back to an uninterrupted workday before you know it. Because the transition back to work can be stressful under the best of circumstances, I recommend returning midweek so you can ease gently into balancing your new working and pumping schedule. Starting on a Wednesday or Thursday gives you a few days to figure out what works best before you dive into your first full work week. Although going back to work while still breastfeeding may seem daunting, many moms have successfully navigated the return to work while maintaining their breastfeeding relationship with their baby.

Current U.S. Breastfeeding and Pumping at Work Regulations

As of 2010, the Fair Labor Standards Act instituted federal protections for breastfeeding moms. The "Break Time for Nursing Mothers" portion of the act requires that employers allow every new mother who is an hourly, non-exempt employee "reasonable break time… to express breast milk for her nursing child for one year after the child's birth each time such employee has need to express the milk." Employers are also required to provide "a place, other than a bathroom, that is shielded from view and free from intrusion from coworkers and the public, which may be used by an employee to express breast milk." Note that employers with fewer than 50 employees are not required to offer nursing mothers break time if the time away would cause "undue hardship." Most states have their own laws related to breastfeeding, which may be more favorable than the federal requirements for moms returning to work. These laws may include providing break time for pumping for exempt employees or for employees working for companies with fewer than 50 employees, provisions for pumping beyond one year, and financial compensation for pumping break time. Many employers realize that supporting breastfeeding mothers can benefit the company, since breastfeeding moms miss less work as a result of staying home with sick children and employees feel happier and better supported, prompting less employee turnover. For more information on the current United States federal laws, visit the US Department of Labor website at www.dol.gov/whd/nursingmothers/. For information on your particular state's current laws, visit the National Conference of State Legislatures website at www.ncsl.org/research/health/breastfeeding -state-laws.aspx.

Consult with Your Employer Ahead of Time

Before you return to work, discuss expectations with your supervisor (and/or someone in your human resources department) regarding when, where, and how often you will be pumping during the workday. I recommend having this conversation as far in advance of your return as you can. It's always nice when another employee has paved the way for you by educating your employer on the law. However, if you are the first employee who will be pumping at work, ask where you will be pumping and what amenities, if any, will be provided. In a perfect scenario, you will have a designated private mothers' room, complete with a comfortable chair, a sink for washing pump parts, and a refrigerator to store pumped milk. However, don't be surprised if all you get is an empty room with an outlet to plug in your pump. You'll also want to discuss the amount of time you will need to pump during your workday and whether your employer will compensate you for this break time. Some women use their regular break times to pump, which are often paid. When figuring out how much time you'll need, don't forget to allow extra time for walking to your pumping location, setting up your pump, cleaning your pump parts, storing the milk, and returning to your work space. This might take 30 minutes per pump session, including the recommended 15 minutes of pumping.

Pumping in Progress!

One mom's employer was so supportive of her pumping at work that her boss made a sign for her to hang on the door of the pump room that said "Pumping in Progress!" You can bet that no one (especially a male coworker) was going to barge in and interrupt the pumping process. This sign gave her the support and privacy she needed to relax and successfully pump breastmilk for her baby.

EQUIPMENT YOU'LL NEED FOR PUMPING AT WORK

Breast Pump

The majority of moms bring their own personal, double electric breast pump to work each day. A double electric pump enables you to pump both breasts simultaneously, minimizing the time away from work as well as maximizing your milk output. Some large employers offer a multi-user hospital-grade breast pump for employees to use at work. In this case, moms only need to bring their pump parts and tubing. The advantage of a hospital-grade pump is that it removes milk efficiently in a short amount of time. Additionally, if your employer supplies one, you won't need to transport your pump to and from work each day.

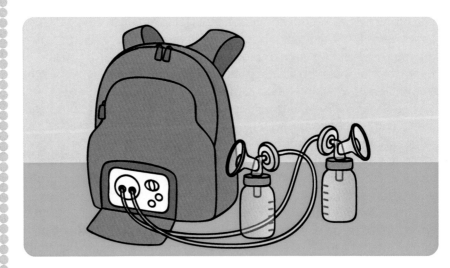

Bottles or Milk Storage Bags

You will need a container in which to collect and store breastmilk at work. Most pumps come with bottles to collect milk while pumping. You can keep the milk in these bottles, but you will then need a set for each pumping session. Many moms collect milk in bottles and then transfer it to breastmilk storage bags. Some bags have an adapter that fits onto the pump parts so you can pump milk directly into the bags, eliminating the need to wash bottles after pumping. Just make sure to look for a breastmilk storage bag brand that uses BPA-free plastic. After expressing, you can store your milk in a refrigerator or a cooler bag with ice for up to 24 hours. If you are storing milk in a communal fridge, you might want to put the milk inside an opaque bag for privacy.

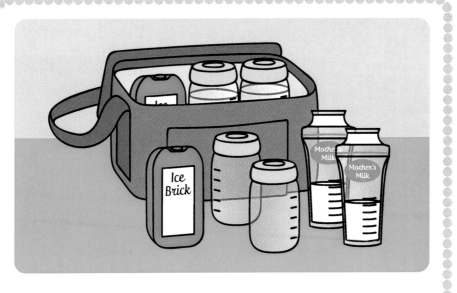

Hands-Free Pumping Bra

Many moms like to use a hands-free pumping bra while pumping at work so they can use their hands to massage their breasts (to maximize milk output) or to check email, make phone calls, or do other work-related tasks. My favorite hands-free pumping bras are made by Simple Wishes (www.simplewishes.com). A sports bra with holes cut into the front to hold the breast shields works just as well. Disposable breast pads placed inside your bra are useful for drying up any milk that might leak from your breasts when you are done pumping.

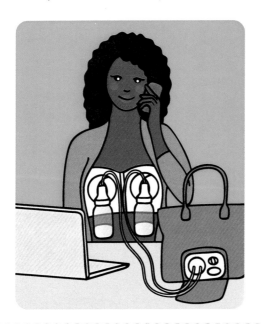

Cleaning Pump Parts

After pumping, wash all pump parts with warm soapy water and let them air dry. This includes the flanges, bottles, and valves/membranes. It's important to completely separate the valve from the flange for cleaning to avoid mold growth. There is no need to wash the tubing, since only air moves through it. To save time, many moms purchase extra flanges and bottles, so they don't need to clean their pump parts in between pumping sessions while at work. Another time-saving option is to use microwavable steam clean bags or wipes to clean pump parts in between uses, which also cuts down on cleaning time.

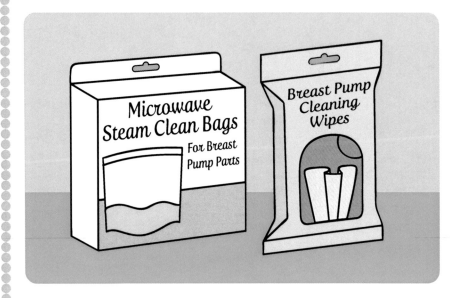

How Often to Pump

To protect your milk supply while you are away from your baby, pump both breasts at the same time for fifteen minutes approximately every three hours. You don't need to try to time pumping with exactly when your baby is eating. There will be days when you can't get out of a meeting at exactly the three-hour mark. Just try to pump as soon as you can. Your breasts probably will be telling you it's time to pump, too! Although your body will get used to pumping during the work week, you can breastfeed your baby on demand when you are with her, even if the feeding times do not correlate exactly with your pump times at work.

Pumping Schedule

Your pumping schedule will depend on the timing of your first feeding of the day, your commute time, and the number of hours you expect to be away from your baby. Some moms find it convenient to pump in the car during their commute, using a car adapter. You can decide what works best for you and your family. For a professional who works an eight-to-five workday in an office, a pumping schedule might look something like this.

Sample Schedule for Pumping at Work

6:00 a.m.	Breastfeed baby upon waking
9:00 a.m.	Double pump for 15 minutes during commute or at work
12:00 p.m.	Double pump for 15 minutes at lunchtime
3:00 p.m.	Double pump for 15 minutes at work
6:00 p.m.	Breastfeed baby upon reuniting and through the evening

Introducing a Bottle

Adjusting to a back-to-work routine can be stressful enough without worrying if your baby will take a bottle while you are gone. To avoid this anxiety, introduce a bottle to your baby at least a few weeks ahead of time, if you haven't already. The best time to introduce a bottle is when your baby is between four and six weeks old, after breastfeeding is established. If your baby has not yet taken a bottle, or is reluctant to take one from you, try having your partner bottle-feed her. Offer at least two or three bottles each week before returning to work to keep your baby interested. If your baby refuses a bottle before your return to work, see the section on bottle refusal on page 68.

Paced Bottle Feeding

The most respectful and least stressful way to bottle feed a baby is using the paced bottle feeding method. With paced bottle feeding, your baby has more control over how fast the milk flows, allowing her to eat at her own pace and avoid tummy discomfort after feedings. Paced bottle feeding also decreases baby's frustration at the breast.

If she gets accustomed to a quick flow from the bottle, she may become fussy during breastfeeding when the milk flows more slowly and sporadically. Lastly, if baby consumes milk too quickly, she may continue to show hunger cues, even if she isn't really hungry, because she did not suckle long enough to fulfill her suck need. Ideally, bottle feedings should take about five minutes per ounce of milk offered. To pace a bottle feeding, hold your baby upright and the bottle horizontal. Let the milk fill the nipple about halfway. Continue holding the bottle horizontally throughout the feeding, allowing your baby to pause when she desires. This lets her pace the feeding and prevents her from drinking too quickly. Although she will take in some air during the feeding, you can easily alleviate any potential discomfort by burping her halfway through and at the end of the feeding. For additional information on Paced Bottle Feeding, see page 85.

Preparing Your Caregiver

It will be important to educate your caregiver about pacing bottle feedings and appropriate amounts of breastmilk to offer. Caregivers at daycare centers may have a lot of babies to feed and may resist using paced bottle feeding because of the amount of time it takes. However, it's important to protect your breastfeeding relationship by making sure your baby is fed using this method. Most babies will eat between one and 1.5 ounces of milk per hour while away from mom. Given this guideline, your caregiver can offer a three- to four-ounce bottle, every three hours. If you have a large milk supply, your baby may be getting more than one ounce per hour when breastfeeding. In this case, you may want to provide several three- to four-ounce bottles as well as a few one- to two-ounce bottles. That way, your caregiver can offer a smaller amount if your baby is not satisfied after three or four ounces or wants a snack just before you arrive for pickup. If possible, breastfeed when you arrive at your child's daycare to prompt your body to create antibodies for whatever germs are in the daycare environment. These antibodies will be present in your breastmilk and will help your baby fight off the germs she will inevitably be exposed to.

Maximizing Output from the Pump

Many of the factors that can cause a decrease in milk supply are also consistent with returning to work. These include stress, lack of sleep, lack of adequate fluids or nutrition, and pumping instead of breastfeeding. It's important to have realistic expectations about the amount of breastmilk you will be able to pump for your baby while at work. The amount of milk you express using the pump is almost always less than the amount your baby gets when breastfeeding. Releasing milk from your breasts, called letdown, is a hormonal process that can be challenging for some moms when their babies are not with them. To maximize pumping output, try developing a relaxing habit or ritual before you start to pump, time permitting. This might be sitting quietly, doing some deep breathing, drinking a glass of water or a warm cup of tea, or listening to relaxing music. Some moms look at pictures or watch videos of their babies before and/or during a pumping session to help increase the milk flow by triggering a hormonal response.

Ways to encourage a letdown before and during pumping include:

- Create a relaxing ritual that you repeat each time, before pumping
- Warm the flanges before pumping
- Shake and/or massage breasts in a circular motion
- Use a comb to lightly stroke breasts from chest to areola
- Smell your baby's clothing or blanket
- Look at pictures and/or videos of your baby

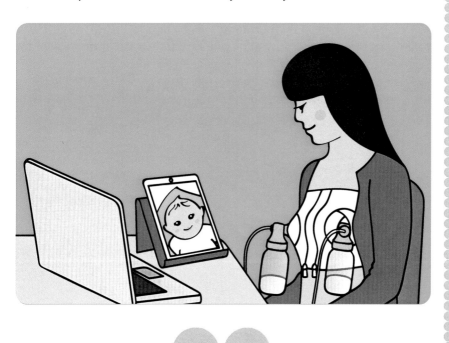

Once your milk starts to flow, if you are wearing a hands-free pumping bra, you can use your hands to continue to massage your breasts while pumping. This may also help to yield more milk. For more information, see the section on Hands-On Pumping on page 81. Time allowing, many moms are able to hand express even more milk once they finish pumping. If you are having trouble pumping enough milk for your baby, see the section on Low Milk Supply on page 74. Note that your milk supply may decrease if you are not having at least eight breast stimulations (either breastfeeding or pumping) in a 24 hour period.

Weaning from the Pump

At some point you will decide to reduce the number of pumping sessions or stop pumping at work altogether, even if you are still breastfeeding when you and your baby are together. Amazingly, you can program your body to have milk available for your baby only when you are with her, such as in the morning and in the evening. Anytime you change the demand for milk, it is important to do so slowly to avoid plugged ducts and mastitis. Wean from one pumping session at a time. Start by reducing the amount of time you pump during a particular pumping session by half. Continue pumping for this decreased amount of time during that pumping session for about three days. Then drop the pumping session altogether. Manage any fullness or engorgement by manually expressing just enough milk so you feel comfortable. Continue this process for all of your regular pumping times until you are completely done pumping or have dropped the desired number of pumping sessions.

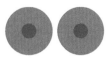

CHAPTER 11
INTRODUCING SOLID FOOD AND WEANING

Introducing solids is essentially the first step in weaning, although you may go on to breastfeed for months or even years. Learning to eat solid food is a gradual process. At first, it's more of a sensory experience than a nutritional one, as your baby explores new tastes and textures with her mouth and tongue. As she learns this new skill, breastfeeding will continue to meet the majority of her nutritional needs. By her first birthday, this will change and solid foods will meet the majority of her nutritional needs.

Introducing Solids

Your pediatrician will recommend the appropriate time to start offering solid foods to your baby, usually when she is between four and six months old. You can also watch for signs that your baby is ready for solids.

Signs your baby is ready for solids:

- Sitting up with support
- Being able to move head and neck easily
- Showing interest in your food while you are eating
- Reaching for your food during meals

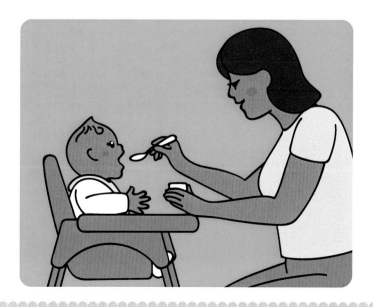

You will start by offering food once a day, so choose a time that is most convenient for you. Offer your baby one or two tablespoons of mashed or puréed food with a small, soft spoon. If you have extra breastmilk, you can mix a little in with the mashed food. It will take time for your baby to learn to move soft food from the front of her mouth to the back so she can swallow. Don't be surprised if little food actually makes it to her tummy, and most ends up on her face or the floor. She will enjoy exploring the different flavors and textures with her tongue, which is all part of the learning process. It's important to introduce only one food at a time. Wait about three days before offering another food to allow time for any potential reaction to reveal itself. This would indicate that your baby may have an allergy or sensitivity to that particular food. Because the number of calories she gets from food will be low initially, breastfeed before offering solids each time, to ensure that your baby is getting enough calories while also protecting your milk supply.

Examples of first soft foods:

- Mashed banana
- Mashed avocado
- Mashed sweet potato

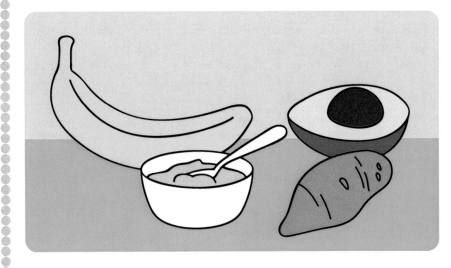

Once your baby has gotten used to mashed or puréed foods and can use her fingers to pick up small objects, you can start offering bite-sized portions of whatever food you are eating, with some exceptions (see below). Eventually your baby will be eating three meals and at least two snacks per day, typically by her first birthday.

Examples of first bite-sized foods:

• Cut up pieces of cooked vegetables
• Cut up pieces of fruit
• Small pieces of well-cooked pasta
• Small pieces of whatever you are eating

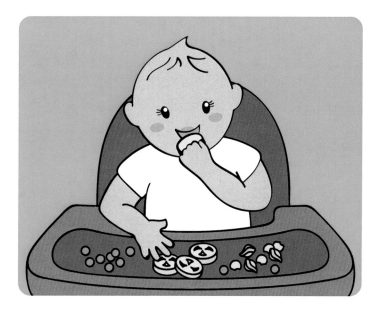

Foods to Avoid

Some foods are not recommended before baby's first birthday for safety reasons. These include honey, which can cause botulism in babies under one year old, and hard foods like hot dogs, whole grapes, and raw vegetables, which are all choking hazards. Allergies to foods such as peanuts and shellfish also may be a concern. Discuss possible allergy issues with your pediatrician. As your baby gets bigger and learns to use her teeth, she will be able to enjoy a larger variety of foods. When your baby shakes her head or turns away, she is telling you that she doesn't like the food you offered or that she is done eating. Most babies will need to try a food several times before they decide whether they like it or not.

Weaning

The decision about when to start weaning your baby is extremely personal and should be based on your individual desires and not on the expectations of your family, friends, or society. If for any reason you wean sooner than you'd like or sooner than you think you should, remember that any amount of breastmilk you provide is a gift to your baby. Don't feel guilty about deciding to wean at any point along your breastfeeding journey. If you are still breastfeeding long after your initial goal or longer than others think you should, you can feel good knowing that you are providing continued nutritional, immunological, and emotional benefits, regardless of your baby's age.

AAP and WHO Recommendations

The American Academy of Pediatrics (AAP) recommends "exclusive breastfeeding for about 6 months, followed by continued breastfeeding as complementary foods are introduced, with continuation of breastfeeding for 1 year or longer as mutually desired by mother and infant."

Similarly, the World Health Organization (WHO) states, "Exclusive breastfeeding is recommended up to 6 months of age, with continued breastfeeding along with appropriate complementary foods up to two years of age or beyond."

Common reasons for weaning:

- Feeling ready for more independence or time away from baby
- Repeated breast infections or persistent painful latch *
- Returning to work
- Pregnancy or desire to get pregnant
- Nursing strike
- Repeated biting

*If the latch remains painful after the first few weeks despite correct positioning, you may want to have your baby evaluated for a tongue or lip tie if you haven't already done so (see page 66.)

Not Ready to Wean

One mom shared with me that although her initial goal was to breastfeed her 16-month-old son for one year, she had no plans to wean him anytime soon. She said she was proud of how hard she had worked to master this skill and that she and her son were both still really enjoying it. She planned to continue to appreciate the experience one day at a time and felt confident she would know when to begin weaning.

Parent-Led Weaning

If you want to wean when your baby is less than one year old, you'll probably lead the process, since most babies do not self-wean before then. Ideally, the weaning process should be gradual for both physical and emotional reasons. Some moms take weeks or even months to fully wean their babies. Because your body has been programmed to continue making milk, it's important to slowly reduce the number of times you breastfeed each day to allow your body to adjust gradually to the new demand. Abrupt weaning can be dangerous and painful, causing plugged ducts or mastitis. The safest approach is to drop no more than one breastfeeding session every few days. Don't begin the weaning process during a potentially stressful time, such as when your baby is ill or teething, has a new caregiver, has a new baby sibling, or during any other major life changes.

How to Wean

Start by dropping one breastfeeding session, which can be either the one that is most convenient for you or the one your baby seems least interested in. Offer your baby a bottle or cup in place of the breastfeeding session. Babies younger than one year should get previously pumped breastmilk, formula, or donor milk. Your breasts will probably feel quite full during this regular feeding time for a few days as your body adjusts to the new schedule. Manage any fullness by manually expressing just enough milk to help you feel comfortable. If you have an abundant milk supply, you may need to use an electric pump to gradually wean from breastfeeding. Pump for only about five minutes or until you feel comfortable. Continue to drop one breastfeeding session no sooner than every few days as your body adjusts. Many moms keep the first morning feeding and/or the bedtime feeding and may continue to breastfeed once or twice a day for as long as they are both still enjoying it. This is called partial weaning. When you are ready to drop the final breastfeeding session, have your partner offer your baby a cup or bottle instead, preferably not in the same place where you typically breastfeed.

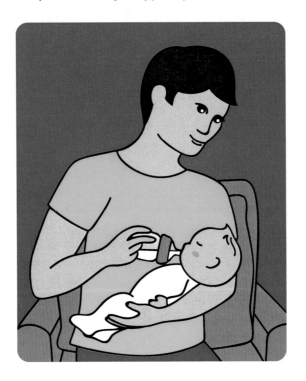

Baby/Child-Led Weaning

Some moms wait until their baby or child shows signs of being ready to wean. If your baby is older than one year, you can offer cow's milk or water in a cup or bottle in place of breastfeeding. Weaning an older baby or child may happen abruptly if she suddenly decides that she no longer wants to breastfeed. However, the process is typically more gradual, as she becomes more interested in eating solid foods and playing with her toys. If you feel ready to wean and you want your baby to control the pace of the weaning process, you can stop offering your breast and wait for her to initiate breastfeeding. This is sometimes referred to as "don't offer, don't refuse."

If you are ready to wean but want your baby to control how quickly the process happens, try some of these suggestions:

- Distract her when she asks to breastfeed.
- Agree to breastfeed but postpone the start time (she may forget she asked).
- Don't uncover your breasts in front of her.
- Don't sit down in the spot where you usually nurse.
- Create a new routine during breastfeeding times (go on a playdate or park visit).
- Offer a new drink or snack during usual breastfeeding times.
- Agree to breastfeed only at home but not in public.
- Breastfeed only when distractions aren't working.

Because your body has gotten used to a predictable routine of breastfeeding, your breasts may feel full during a missed feeding. Manage fullness or discomfort by manually expressing just enough milk to allow you to feel comfortable. If necessary, revisit engorgement treatment options in Chapter 6.

Supporting Your Baby or Child Through Weaning

Depending on how old your child is, she may not be as enthusiastic about weaning as you are. It will be especially important to support your older baby emotionally through this process. Breastfeeding is often a strong bonding experience and many older babies associate breastfeeding with emotional connection. Give her lots of affection and attention during non-breastfeeding times so she knows that breastfeeding is not the only way you show your love. Replace breastfeeding with other forms of nurturing and affection such as reading books while cuddling.

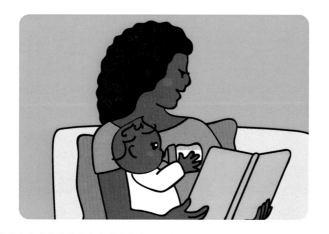

Best-Laid Plans

I remember when my son was 15 months old and I was breastfeeding him only once a day before bedtime. I had an upcoming girls' weekend trip planned and decided it would be the perfect opportunity to drop that last feeding. My husband gave him his milk before bedtime without any problem and I had a great time with my friends. However, when I got back from the trip, I felt a longing to breastfeed again. I didn't want the trip to be the deciding factor in when I chose to wean. I nursed him to sleep for another week and then was able to completely drop that last feeding.

Return of Menses

If your period hasn't yet returned, it will likely resume at some point during or after the weaning process. Some women get a period as early as six weeks postpartum while others don't begin menstruating again until their baby is completely weaned. It is not uncommon to experience a dip in milk supply just before or during your period. Taking a calcium and magnesium supplement a few weeks before your period begins can help prevent this temporary dip. The recommended dosage is 1,500 mg. of calcium and 750 mg. of magnesium divided into three doses per day (500 mg. of calcium and 250 mg. of magnesium per dose). Continue taking these supplements through the first few days of your period each month.

Milk Drying Up

Depending on how long you breastfeed, it can take a while for the milk in your breasts to completely dry up. The longer you breastfeed, the longer it will take. You may be able to manually express some milk for months after you have completely weaned your baby. It's best to avoid breast stimulation during this time to encourage your milk supply to dry up completely.

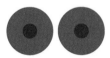

If you are no longer breastfeeding and are still experiencing fullness or lumpiness in your breasts, try these methods:

- Drink sage or peppermint tea.
- Eat mints with peppermint oil.
- Place cold green cabbage leaves inside your bra (see instructions on page 56.)
- Take medicine that dries up mucous membranes (e.g., Sudafed).

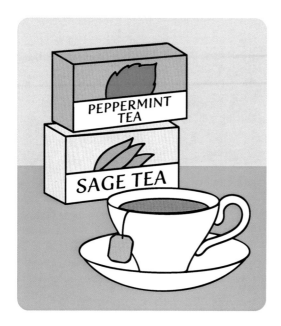

Emotional Side of Weaning

Don't be surprised if you feel a little sad or depressed during or after the weaning process. Your hormone levels will be fluctuating and you may miss the bonding time you shared with your baby. Some moms even experience symptoms of postpartum depression during or directly after the weaning process. For more information about postpartum depression, see Chapter 5.

I hope you feel proud of yourself for mastering the art of breastfeeding and giving your baby the best possible nutrition, using your own body. Breastfeeding provides a strong foundation of emotional connection. However, you will have no shortage of opportunities to continue to bond and connect with your baby, throughout childhood and beyond.

ACKNOWLEDGEMENTS

Writing *Latch Baby* has not been a solo endeavor. I have been lucky to have the support of a wonderful community, and I would like to extend my deepest gratitude to

…all of the parents who so graciously invited me into their homes at such a precious time to help them learn to nourish their babies. You have all taught me so much and it's been a privilege and an honor to support you throughout your breastfeeding experience.

… my illustrator, Bridget Halberstadt, for creating our "latch" baby and bringing it to life through all of the beautiful illustrations in the book. I have enjoyed working with you for over twenty years and I look forward to our next project.

…my editor, Audrey Kalman. I cannot believe I had the good fortune to find an editor who is also a birth doula and breastfeeding educator within my writing group! It was serendipitous, for sure. You have been such a pleasure to work with. Thank you for your fine editing skills and valuable suggestions.

…my cousin, Robyn Crane, who generously shared her wealth of knowledge as an author. This book would not have been completed without your encouragement.

…my beta readers and dear friends, Lisa Stavros and Lexie Munevar. Thank you so much for taking the time to read ALL of the chapters. Your feedback was invaluable to me.

…my best friend, Wendy Trento. Thank you for your unconditional love, support, and endless interest in my latest project.

…my friend and lactation colleague, Sarah Karanian. Your enthusiasm for my lactation ventures has given me so much strength.

…my mentor and friend, Sheila Janakos. Thank you for sharing your amazing wealth of knowledge with me.

Last, but certainly not least, I'd like to thank my family, particularly my husband Dave and my children, Anna and Aaron. Your support and encouragement for this project has warmed my heart. I only hope this book is half as successful as you expect it to be. Thanks also to my pups, Nala and Ellie, for keeping me company while writing. I love you all.

REFERENCES

American Academy of Pediatrics. "AAP Reaffirms Breastfeeding Guidelines." February 27, 2012. Accessed Jan. 5, 2019. www.aap.org/en-us/about-the-aap/aap-press-room/Pages/AAP-Reaffirms-Breastfeeding-Guidelines.aspx

American Academy of Pediatrics. "Infant Food and Feeding." Accessed February 23, 2019. www.aap.org/en-us/advocacy-and-policy/aap-health-initiatives/HALF-Implementation-Guide/Age-Specific-Content/Pages/Infant-Food-and-Feeding.aspx

Ask Dr. Sears. "Average Breastfed Baby Weight Gain." Accessed October 12, 2018. www.askdrsears.com/topics/feeding-eating/breastfeeding/faqs/how-much-weight-will-my-breastfeeding-baby-gain

Baby Connect. Accessed December 6, 2018. www.babyconnect.com

Baby Tracker. Accessed December 6, 2018. www.nighp.com/babytracker/

Baby Wearing International. "What is Babywearing?" Accessed November 1, 2018. www.babywearinginternational.org/what-is-babywearing/

BFAR-Breastfeeding After Breast and Nipple Surgeries. Information and Support. Accessed January 3, 2019. https://www.bfar.org/index.shtml

Biological Nurturing. "Laid back breastfeeding." Accessed August 6, 2019. www.biologicalnurturing.com

CDC. Centers for Disease Control and Prevention. "Proper Storage and Preparation of Breast Milk." Accessed October 15, 2018. www.cdc.gov/breastfeeding/recommendations/handling_breastmilk.htm

CDC. Centers for Disease Control and Prevention. "Sudden Unexpected Infant Death and Sudden Infant Death Syndrome." Accessed March 15,, 2018. www.cdc.gov/breastfeeding/recommendations/handling_breastmilk.htm

DONA International. Accessed December 1, 2017. www.dona.org

Eats on Feets. Accessed February 16, 2018. www.eatsonfeets.org

Einhorn, Amy. *The Fourth Trimester*. New York: Crown Publishers, 2001.

Haakaa USA. Accessed July 6, 2017. www.haakaausa.com

HealthCare. Health Benefits & Coverage. "Breastfeeding Benefits." Accessed November 5, 2018. www.healthcare.gov/coverage/breast-feeding-benefits/

Healthychildren. "Alcohol & Breast Milk." Accessed February 8, 2019. www.healthychildren.org/English/ages-stages/baby/breastfeeding/Pages/Alcohol-Breast-Milk.aspx

Huggins, Kathleen. *The Nursing Mother's Companion.* 7th ed. Beverly, MA: Harvard Common Press, 2015.

IBLCE International Board of Lactation Consultant Examiners. Accessed March 20, 2017. www.iblce.org

ILCA International Lactation Consultant Association. Accessed April 2, 2017. www.ilca.org

Kangaroo Mother Care. "Kangaroo Mother Care for every preterm and fullterm baby." Accessed September 16, 2018. www.kangaroomothercare.com

Kindred Bravely. Accessed June 5, 2018. www.kindredbravely.com

Lauwers, Judith, and Anna Swisher. *Counseling the Nursing Mother.* 4th ed. Burlington, MA: Jones Bartlett Learning, 2005.

La Leche League International. Accessed October 24, 2017. www.llli.org

Mommy Meds. "Breastfeeding," Accessed October 20, 2018. www.mommymeds.com/breastfeeding

My Milkies. Accessed November 3, 2018. www.mymilkies.com

My Brest Friend. Accessed July 2, 2017. www.mybrestfriend.com

Newman, Jack and Teresa Pitman. *Dr. Jack Newman's Guide to Breastfeeding.* Toronto, Canada: Pinter & Martin, 2014.

Postpartum Support International. "Pregnancy & Postpartum Mental Health Overview." Accessed January 5, 2019. www.postpartum.net/learn-more/pregnancy-postpartum-mental-health/

SeePPD. "Symptoms of Postpartum Depression". Accessed January 5, 2019. www.seeppd.com/signs-of-postpartum-depression/symptoms/

Simple Wishes. Accessed November 12, 2017. www.simplewishes.com

Shortall, Jessica. *Work. Pump. Repeat.* New York, NY: Abrams Books, 2015

Stanford Children's Health. "Newborn-Sleep Patterns". Accessed October 11, 2018. www.stanfordchildrens.org/en/topic/default?id=newborn-sleep-patterns-90-P02632

Stanford University Newborn Nursery. "Hand Expression of Breastmilk." Accessed October 1, 2018. med.stanford.edu/newborns/professional-education/breastfeeding/abcs-of-breastfeeding/hand-expression-of-breast-milk.html

Tongue Tie from Confusion to Clarity. "Breastfeeding with a Tongue Tie Baby." Accessed August 8, 2018. www.tonguetie.net/breastfeeding/

Tummy Time! Method. "The Tummy Time Method." Accessed December 18, 2018. www.tummytimemethod.com/tummytimetrade-method.html

United States Department of Labor. "Break Time for Nursing Mothers". Accessed January 20, 2019. www.dol.gov/whd/nursingmothers/

University of Wisconsin Integrative Health, Department of Family Medicine and Community Health. "Supplement Sampler." Accessed November 15, 2018. www.fammed.wisc.edu/files/webfm-uploads/documents/outreach/im/ss_galactogogues.pdf

Upspring Baby. Accessed December 11, 2018. www.upspringbaby.com

Walker, Marsha. *Breastfeeding Management for the Clinician*. 4th ed. Burlington, MA: Jones Bartlett Learning, 2017.

Watson Genna, Catherine. *Supporting Sucking Skills in Breastfeeding Infants*. 2nd ed. Burlington, MA: Jones Bartlett Learning, 2013.

Wiessinger, Diane, Diana West, and Teresa Pitman. *The Womanly Art of Breastfeeding*. 8th ed. New York: Ballantine Books, 2010.

World Health Organization. "10 Facts on Breastfeeding." Accessed February 1, 2019. www.who.int/features/factfiles/breastfeeding/facts/en/

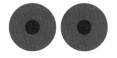

INDEX

Made in United States
North Haven, CT
02 June 2022

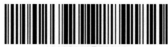

19803070R00066